the fast beach diet

Previous titles in the *FastDiet* series:

The FastDiet: Lose Weight, Stay Healthy, and Live Longer with the Simple Secret of Intermittent Fasting

The FastDiet Cookbook: 150 Delicious, Calorie-Controlled Meals to Make Your Fasting Days Easy

FastExercise: The Simple Secret of High-Intensity Training

the fast beach diet

The Super-Fast Plan to Lose Weight and Get in Shape in Just Six Weeks

MIMI SPENCER

with a foreword by
Dr. Michael Mosley

ATRIA PAPERBACK

NEW YORK   LONDON   TORONTO   SYDNEY   NEW DELHI

ATRIA PAPERBACK
A Division of Simon & Schuster, Inc.
1230 Avenue of the Americas
New York, NY 10020

Copyright © 2014 by Mimi Spencer

Originally published in 2014 in Great Britain by Short Books.

All rights reserved, including the right to reproduce this book or portions thereof in any form whatsoever. For information, address Atria Books Subsidiary Rights Department, 1230 Avenue of the Americas, New York, NY 10020.

First Atria Paperback edition June 2014

ATRIA PAPERBACK and colophon are trademarks of Simon & Schuster, Inc.

For information about special discounts for bulk purchases, please contact Simon & Schuster Special Sales at 1-866-506-1949 or business@simonandschuster.com.

The Simon & Schuster Speakers Bureau can bring authors to your live event. For more information or to book an event contact the Simon & Schuster Speakers Bureau at 1-866-248-3049 or visit our website at www.simonspeakers.com.

Manufactured in the United States of America

10   9   8   7   6   5   4   3   2   1

Library of Congress Cataloging-in-Publication Data

Spencer, Mimi.
  The fastbeach diet : the super-fast plan to lose weight and get in shape in just six weeks / Mimi Spencer ; with a foreword by Dr. Michael Mosley.
    pages   cm
  title: Fast beach diet
  1. Reducing diets. 2. Weight loss. I. Mosley, Michael - writer of preface. II. Title. III. Title: Fast beach diet.
  RM222.2.S6747 2014
  613.2'5—dc23   2014016977

ISBN 978-1-4767-9039-8
ISBN 978-1-4767-9040-4 (ebook)

Contents

Foreword

The Fast Way to Better Health

Intermittent Fasting is, without doubt, one of the hottest new approaches to weight loss on the planet. When *The FastDiet* was published in January 2013, Mimi and I could never have imagined the response it would get. It quickly became an international phenomenon, and has since been embraced by celebrities like Beyoncé and Benedict Cumberbatch ("You have to, for *Sherlock*"). *One Foot in the Grave* star Richard Wilson told a newspaper that he had lost 12 pounds on the diet in just five weeks. "The great thing is that the fasting days are tough but you know that the next day you can eat." Even the slim new Chancellor of the Exchequer, George Osborne, is rumored to be on it.

I am passionate about IF because I find the science compelling and because there is such good evidence of potential health benefits. I am also convinced by the dramatic effects it has had on my own body. By way of background, for those of you who have not read the original book, two years ago I was an overweight middle-aged man, weighing in at around 185 pounds, with a 36-inch waist. I was mildly embarrassed about the spare tire round my gut, but not embarrassed enough to do anything about it.

Then I went to my doctor with a minor complaint and as part of the examination she suggested I have a routine blood test. When the results came back she told me that I was a type 2 diabetic, with a fasting glucose of around 7.2 mmol/l. This was a nasty shock as my father had passed away at a relatively early age; when he died he was suffering from a range of diseases, including type 2 diabetes, heart failure, prostate cancer, and what I suspect was early dementia.

Rather than start on medication, I began researching alternative approaches and came across IF. I decided to make a documentary on the subject; in the course of making the film *Eat, Fast, Live Longer*, I tried various different forms of IF, ranging from doing five days of almost total calorie restriction to alternate-day fasting (where you cut your calories every other day). Eventually I settled on a pattern I found easy to stick to, which I called the 5:2 diet.

On a Monday and a Thursday I ate a quarter of my normal calorie intake, going down from around 2,400 to 600 calories a day. In 12 weeks on this diet I lost nearly 20 pounds and 4 inches off my waist. My body fat went down from 28% to 21%. My blood glucose fell to healthy levels. I also began to sleep better (I lost fat around my neck and stopped snoring).

I then began combining the IF with an intermittent exercise regimen (FastExercise) and soon began to see the beginnings of a six-pack. I can now fit into a suit I haven't worn for 30 years.

As our website testifies, this is an experience that has been replicated thousands of times over. We now have feedback from countless people who have embarked on the 5:2 FastDiet and found it to be positively life changing.

So why has Mimi written a new book? Well, the original book laid out the science behind IF and gave useful tips on how to do it. What it didn't do was produce a structured program, one that would ensure fat loss over a comparatively short period of time. *The FastBeach Diet* is an adjunct, if you like, designed to complement the original *FastDiet*—a short-term, faster solution for those of you who perhaps have a fat-loss deadline to meet.

The original book also made very little reference to exercise. Although studies show that low intensity exercise, like jogging, is unlikely to lead to weight loss (people tend to compensate by eating more), there is plenty of evidence that a combination of calorie restriction and exercise will lead to more sustained weight loss than either done alone. *The FastBeach Diet* includes useful sections on how to get fitter and better toned in just a few minutes a day.

Best of all, Mimi has produced a range of new and tasty recipes for your Fast Days. I have begun to work my way through them and can testify that they are full of flavor as well as hunger-killing fiber and protein.

I greatly enjoyed reading this book and learned something new from doing so. I hope you do too.

Dr. Michael Mosley

Chapter 1

The FastDiet Revisited . . .
and an Invitation
to the Beach

"A year from now, you will wish you started today."

There are many good reasons to start the FastDiet. You may be inspired by your sister or your best friend, your dad or your doctor. You may have decided you want to cut your risk of age-related disease. You may want to reduce your cholesterol, boost your brain, improve your mood, lower your blood pressure, lengthen your life.

Or you may just want to look good in a swimsuit.

I say "just." But looking good and (more importantly) feeling good about your body is no mere vanity project. It can have a real emotional impact on a life. I'm reminded of one FastDieter who told me that, after years of fruitless yo-yo dieting, six months of 5:2 had given her enough body confidence to go to the local pool and swim with her young daughter for the first time ever. That's not vanity. It's the glorious stuff of life.

Not long ago, a magazine survey found that women think about their bodies every 15 minutes (which is, apparently, more than men think about sex). There are times of the year, of course, when we put ourselves under greater scrutiny still. On the beach, in summer, in our shorts and bikinis, we think about the shape we're in even more often—a constant background hum, the helicopter moaning overhead. Men may not go on about it quite as much, but they tend to be just as aware as T-shirt weather creeps up to ambush those hibernating pecs and paunches.

So now is the time to act. The beach beckons and this is your call to arms. The most challenging weeks of the year may be looming on the sun-kissed horizon, but that's no reason to bury your head in the sand or collapse into a kaftan for cover. We have a plan. It is called the FastBeach Diet. Think of it as "5:2, the Next Generation." It promises to shake things up, with a wealth of new tips, tricks, and takes to help you break the plateau, make the leap and reboot your 5:2 for summer. In the words of the late, great Janis Joplin, we're gonna try . . . just a little bit harder. But first, let's recap on the original FastDiet—what it is and how it works.

What Is the FastDiet?

It may be radical, but the FastDiet is also wonderfully economical with its rules. I like that *The Times* has called it the "haiku diet"—a pithy, almost poetic agenda. All you really need to know is that:

• You eat normally for five days a week and then, for the other two days, you consume a quarter of your normal calorie intake—around 600 calories for men, 500 for women. So, it is not total "fasting," but a modified version.

- It is not continual fasting, but intermittent. Our experience is that nonconsecutive Fast Days work best, though you can do them back to back if you prefer.

- Most people divide their calorie allowance between breakfast and an evening meal, aiming for a lengthy "fasting window" between meals. But you can skip breakfast and have a more substantial evening meal containing your whole calorie quota if it better suits your day.

- It does matter what you eat on a Fast Day: plan your calorie quota by sticking, as the recipes in chapter 7 do, to the FastDiet mantra: "Mostly Plants and Protein." That way, you'll stay full longer and get adequate nutrients in your diet.

Why 5:2?

In the beginning, Michael tried several different fasting regimens; the one he settled on as the most realistic and sustainable was five days off, two days on, which meant that the majority of the time was spent free from calorie-counting. On this program, in 12 weeks Michael lost more than 20 pounds of body fat and his blood glucose fell to a healthy level. I lost 22 pounds and returned to my pre-motherhood body weight (and, more importantly, shape).

That was only a little over 18 months ago. We're still learning about the true long-term benefits of IF, and we don't, as yet, have a comprehensive account of potential pitfalls, particularly why some people flourish on 5:2 and others may find it harder. It may be that there is no "one size fits all." What we do know is that thousands of people have followed the FastDiet, lost weight, gained health, and found it surprisingly sustainable, effective, and life affirming. New studies are underway and we hope to bring together the latest thinking in a fully updated new edition to be published in 2015.

So Where's the Catch?

Really, there isn't one. The FastDiet, don't forget, is simply a modern take on an ancient idea. Fasting, in one form or another, has been practiced for centuries by most of the great religions, and if done properly seems to be extremely safe. There is no evidence of significant side effects (though some people may experience headaches and constipation, particularly at first; these can generally be prevented by drinking lots of water or calorie-free fluids, such as black coffee and herbal tea, and eating foods rich in fiber).

Indeed, the FastDiet has helped to debunk some of the myths that have developed around the way we eat in the West—for instance that:

• You need to eat whenever you feel hungry.

• Eating every few hours will increase your metabolic rate.

• If you don't eat every few hours your blood sugar will fall and you will feel faint.

None of these widely held beliefs is backed by science. You will discover that short bouts of hunger are manageable and soon pass. Similarly, there is no metabolic advantage to spreading your calories over the day, nor is there any evidence that short periods without food will cause your blood glucose to plunge to seriously low levels. Most nights, don't forget, you happily go 12 hours without eating, and many people feel fine with a late breakfast, especially on a Sunday when the start can be in delicious slow-motion.

Should You Be Skeptical?

Michael and I certainly were. After all, anyone who has ever gone on a conventional diet knows that they are hard work; they may deliver results in the short term, but then life gets in the way—we're soon bored and the weight creeps back on. We've found, however, that the 5:2 FastDiet does work—for exactly the reason that other diets don't: there is none of the boredom, frustration, or serial denial that characterises standard diet plans; eating is still a pleasure; there's no cutting of food groups, no pathologizing of eating. And indeed, even the turbo version laid out here is full of forgiveness, generosity of spirit, and the crucial adaptability required to fit it into a busy life.

A Word on the Benefits of Intermittent Fasting

The reason behind IF—briefly but severely restricting the number of calories you consume—is that it "fools" your body into thinking it is in a potential famine situation and that it needs to switch from go-go mode to maintenance mode. Fasting is the shock that resets the clock. Its many benefits include:

• Fat loss of 1–2 pounds a week

• A reduction in a hormone called IGF-1, which means that you are reducing your risk of a number of age-related diseases

• The switching on of repair genes

• Improvements in cardiovascular health and cholesterol levels

• A rest for your pancreas, boosting the effectiveness of the insulin it produces in response to elevated blood glucose

• Metabolic changes that tweak your body into burning fat and increase its insulin sensitivity; this in turn will reduce your risk of obesity, diabetes, heart disease, and cognitive decline

• Increased levels of neurotrophic factor in the brain, which should make you more cheerful, even when contemplating your summer swimsuit

The FastDiet and Weight Loss

While clinical studies into IF in general, and 5:2 in particular, are still in their early stages, there's a great deal of convincing anecdotal evidence that the approach can be startlingly effective for many people. Anecdote, as Michael often says, makes poor science, but it does tell a story. Many thousands of people have adopted the plan and witnessed significant improvements in their weight, cholesterol, and general health, and have gone on to post their success stories online (we have included just a fraction of these in the testimonials chapter at the back of this book). We regularly meet people on the street and see friends and family who've lost weight and gained health. My father, for instance, has lost 56 pounds over the course of a year on the FastDiet. That's about the weight of an eight-year-old child. I can now get my arms all the way around him when we hug hello. It's a seismic change, and a joy to behold.

HOW FASTING TARGETS FAT

What people sometimes forget in their drive to "lose weight" is what they really want to lose is not weight as such, but fat. Carrying excess fat is not just a bummer on the beach; it's bad for your health. Here's what we know about the effect IF has on fat:

- It achieves a gradual weight loss—and it's almost all fat.
- It increases fat burn. More of the calories you use for fuel during a fast come from fat stores than muscle. A study from Nottingham University[1] found that the proportion of energy obtained from fat rose progressively over 12–72 hours of fasting, until almost all the energy being used was coming from stored fat.
- When we eat, we use the carbohydrates and fat supplied by the food for fuel, instead of tapping into our stored fat reserves. Constant grazing may be what's keeping fat from being burned—and fasting is one way to release it.
- Interestingly, the heavier you are, the more likely it is that fasting will lead to substantial fat loss with muscle being spared.
- A bonus for Intermittent Fasters is that it seems to lead not just to fat loss generally, but specifically to fat loss around the gut—this is the visceral fat and is particularly dangerous because it increases your risk of heart disease and diabetes.
- One reason why it's important to preserve as much muscle mass as possible is that muscle is metabolically active. Lean tissue burns calories, even at rest.

So Why the FastBeach Diet?

The FastDiet's unique selling point seems to be its high level of compliance: we do it and we stick with it because most of the time, we're not thinking about dieting at all. But some fasters want to boost the process at certain times of year. You may be one of those for whom the 5:2 has not proved the magic bullet you hoped for. Others among you may want to nudge yourself off a plateau and budge any reluctant pounds that are hanging on despite your adherence to 5:2.

I've written this book to be used as a primer for the summer holidays; the idea is to start the six-week regimen in May, June, or July, in good time for take off (that's clothes, not planes). The longer, brighter days and fresher produce of late spring and early summer make it an ideal time to embark or improve upon a weight-loss program. And, as we've already established, there's nothing like an approaching bikini—or T-shirt—to make you think twice about that piece of pie.

That said, the principles of the turbo-driven 5:2 diet laid out here are applicable at almost any time of the year. You might like to use its additional hints and ideas if you are preparing to get married, if you have a big event coming up, if you're starting a new phase in your life, if you're ready to lose some baby weight, or if you've had a particularly sedentary and glutonous couple of months (after Christmas perhaps).

You may, of course, be coming to *The FastBeach Diet* cold, without having read or acted upon the original book. This book is an adjunct. Think of it as a boot camp for the 5:2. It is a condensed, modified program of greater intensity with the aim of helping you achieve a reasonable target weight in a six-week period. Note now that on the FastBeach Diet, you will be encouraged to step it up—to get a bit tougher, a bit bolder, with your FastDiet. But this extra commitment is intended to be short-lived. Just a bit more effort. For just six weeks.

Why Six Weeks?

In truth, the six-week figure is fairly arbitrary. I have used my own experience and a 25-year career in the fashion and fitness business, together with what I have learned from many other dieters, to come up with a reasonable period during which I believe the average individual—someone with a little willpower and plenty of good intentions—can commit to and concentrate on a more intense 5:2 regimen. It hinges on attention span and compliance; six weeks should be enough time to see measurable results without boredom setting in. It's also, by happy coincidence, about the length of time we usually give ourselves to prepare mentally and physically for our summer vacations . . . the Six-Week Sprint to the pool.

You may choose to extend the FastBeach Diet, perhaps to two months. But be clear: it is only meant to be a short-term option; afterwards, you should return to the classic FastDiet rules, without undue concern for calories on a non-Fast Day. Remember: it is this flexible and sociable foundation that lends the FastDiet its psychological advantage.

If the FastBeach Diet seems unnecessarily faddish to you, or if you're not keen on a "fast-fix" message, if you treasure the absolute simplicity of the original FastDiet—well, I empathize and understand. Just stick with your original 5:2 FastDiet. This book is aimed at people who want a short-term booster plan to get them from A (the sofa) to B (the beach) by undertaking a reasonable but more vigorous protocol. It's not designed to be a "forever plan" like the 5:2. It's the FastDiet, just a bit faster. So are you in? Here's what to expect . . .

The FastBeach Diet includes:

• A clear six-week plan to encourage fat loss

• Plateau-busting techniques to jump-start the 5:2 and make it work for you

• Mindfulness methods to help you tough out a fast and eat with understanding every day

• Habit-changing ideas to sharpen up on non-Fast Days

• A High Intensity Training (HIT) exercise program for fitness and fat loss, achievable in just a few minutes a day

• Lots of brand-new, calorie-counted summer recipes, with plenty of healthy, speedy ideas for busy days

• Motivation, meal plans, and 5:2 support to rev up your FastDiet and help get you beach fit for summer

When Should You Start?

If you do not have an underlying medical condition, and if you are not an individual for whom fasting is proscribed (see the disclaimer on page 4), then there really is no time like the present. But first, a bit of prep.

Chapter 2

Getting Started

Know Yourself

Weigh In and Plot Your Progress

Before the kickoff, you really need to understand what shape you're in. It's time for a reality check; shrug off the winter layers and see what lies beneath. While noting the aphorism that "good health is not about weight; weight is an indicator of good health," it is worth knowing your current weight, monitoring your progress, and having a target in mind.

- Ideally, use a scale that measures body-fat percentage as well as weight, since what you really want to see is body-fat levels fall. Women tend to have more body fat than men. A man with body fat of more than 25% is considered overweight. For a woman, it's 30%.

- Though not without controversy, the easiest way to gauge which weight category you fall into (healthy, overweight, obese) is by calculating your Body Mass Index (BMI). This is your weight (in pounds) divided by your height (in inches) squared multiplied by 703. Do note that a BMI score takes no account of body type, age, or ethnicity, so it should be treated with informed caution. Still, if you need a number, this is the one to watch.

- Use the BMI equation to calculate an upper and lower limit for your desirable target weight. So, for example, I am 5'7". A normal, healthy BMI is between 18.5 and 24.9, so a reasonable weight for my height would be somewhere between 117 pounds and 158 pounds. This is obviously a fairly wide range: it's up to you to decide what's right and what's possible.

- If you are significantly heavier than your target weight, see your doctor before embarking on the FastBeach Diet. It's important that any weight-loss or exercise program is safe, and heavier individuals should seek medical advice before starting.

- Measure your waist as an indicator of internal "visceral" fat: male or female, ideally your waist should be less than half your height. Most people underestimate their waist size by about two inches because they rely on trouser size. Instead, measure your waist by putting the tape measure around your belly button.

- You may choose to have your blood tested for fasting glucose (an important measure of fitness and predictor of future health), cholesterol, and triglycerides. Your doctor should be able to do this.

Be Realistic

Precipitous weight loss is not advised, so be sensible and choose a target that seems reasonable. Make a plan. Write it down, recognizing that dieters who keep an honest account of what they eat and drink are more likely to lose the pounds and keep them off. Try using the chart included in this book. I suggest weighing yourself twice a week, first thing in the morning, preferably the day after a fast. You might like to use a tracker—the FastBeach Diet app will do this, or try the tracker at www.thefastdiet.co.uk to plot your progress.

Remember, everyone is different. There will almost certainly be fluctuations in your weight. Some weeks, you may achieve impressive weight loss. Others, you may grind to a halt. If you have not been on the FastDiet already, you may find that in the early weeks of the FastBeach Diet your weight drops quite quickly (some of this will be water). What you're looking for is a downward trajectory, with an average weight loss of about 2 pounds a week; but don't get hung up on the day-to-day numbers. Realize that the goal here is HEALTH. Looking good in a swimsuit is nice. But a long and healthy life is so much better.

Prepare Yourself

As 5:2 devotees well know, it's worth spending a little time getting ready for a Fast Day. Don't overthink it, but it does matter that you have at least considered what, how, and when you're likely to eat—not least because we live in an "obesogenic environment" with opportunities to consume calories at every turn. If you are embarking on the six-week FastBeach Diet, here's how to maximize your chances of success . . .

Plan Your Fast Days

- Eliminate illicit food stashes: empty your snack drawer at work; clear the house of junk food. Those cookies may look innocuous, but they're out to trip you up.

- Shop on non-Fast Days, so as not to taunt yourself with undue temptation.

- Stock up on herbal teas and healthy low-calorie drinks (see pages 61–62).

- Remember: if you don't buy it, you can't forage for it, so shop wisely. Buy more fresh vegetables and have them handy.

- Have a clear idea of your favorite Fast Day foods, remembering to embrace Variety and Volume—the double V key to staying fuller longer.

- Make good Fast Day food in advance and have it ready in the freezer. Keep it simple, aiming for flavor without effort (for great recipe ideas, see chapter 7).

- Don't bump into food by accident—if you're in a rush, you'll never make yourself an interesting salad. You'll stop off at the gas station and buy a pack of M&Ms.

- Be flexible—work out your plan according to your needs, the shape of your day, your family, your commitments, your preferences. You may like to eat once, or twice, first thing or last. Some individuals prefer to be told exactly what to eat and when; others like a more informal approach. That's fine. It's enough to simply stick to the basic method—500 or 600 calories a day, with as long a "window without food" as possible, twice a week—and you'll gain the plan's multiple benefits.

Clear the Diary

Begin on a day when you feel strong, purposeful, calm, and committed. Tell friends and family that you're starting the FastBeach Diet: as we'll see, once you make a public commitment, you are much more likely to stick with it. Avoid vacations, holidays, and days when you know food will be the focus. But do keep busy; it's the best way to zip through a Fast Day and on to tomorrow without dwelling too much on the process. Some women may find fasting more challenging on the days preceding a period; we don't yet have any clear human studies on the impact of IF on the menstrual cycle, but if you feel this may be the case for you, perhaps fast on the days following the start of your period, not before.

Clear Your Mind

Not as frivolous as it sounds: the success of your FastBeach Diet will depend largely on getting your mind in gear at the outset. Think positive. Stay strong. Be bold. Have a clear idea of what you want, why you want it, and what the hurdles may be. To help yourself, answer the following questions before you start:

• What's my motivation?

• What's my weakness?

• What's my goal?

Write down the answers and put them somewhere handy—tucked in your wallet, stuffed in the bread box, stuck inside the front door with tape . . . Once you're off the blocks, you may well find, as many FastDieters do, that occasional fasting makes you feel more connected, happier in yourself. There's plenty more on motivation and mindfulness in the pages ahead.

Chapter 3

Your Fast Days in Practice

So. Today's the day. Six weeks until the great reveal. We all do it, don't we? We calculate a reasonable interval between now and the first beach outing, a window of opportunity and diligence that, in theory, should get us swimsuit-ready in a great six-week leap. Women apparently plan to lose an average of 8 pounds before a vacation. The operative word here is "plan." I suspect that the reason everyone looks so despondent in the departure lounge at the airport is that they've all been bitterly disappointed by the scales that very morning. But with the FastBeach Diet, you're stacking the odds in your favor. Stay focused. Stay firm. This, you can do.

Which Days to Choose

It really doesn't matter. It's your life, and you'll know which days will suit you best. Monday is an obvious choice for many, perhaps because it is more manageable, psychologically and practically, to gear yourself up at the beginning of a new week, particularly if it follows a sociable weekend. For that reason, fasters might choose to avoid Saturdays and Sundays, when family lunches and brunches, dinner dates, and parties make calorie cutting a bore. Thursday would then make a sensible second Fast Day, echoing, if such things appeal to you, the teachings of the Prophet Muhammad, who is understood to have fasted the second and fifth days of the week. But be flexible; don't force yourself to fast when it feels wrong. If you're particularly stressed, off-color, tired, or peevish on a day that you have designated a fast, try again another day. Adapt. Do, however, aim for a pattern. That way, over the six-week period, your fasts will become familiar, a low-key habit you accept and embrace.

When to Eat

Go with a timetable that suits you. Some fasters appreciate the convenience and simplicity of a single 500/600-calorie evening meal, allowing them to ignore food entirely for most of the day; some people say they actually feel hungrier during the day if they have breakfast. Having just one meal, as late in the day as possible, will clearly intensify the fast— allowing your body a longer period in which to be in a fasted state. Others prefer to eat breakfast and then avoid food for a fasting window of around 12 hours until dinner.

Since it is the fasted state that is so beneficial to us, eating lots of small meals is likely to significantly reduce the benefits, particularly if you graze on carbohydrates. Mark Mattson at the National Institute on Aging agrees that eating the 500/600 calories at one meal is better than eating several smaller meals over the course of the day. It is, however, only "better" if you actually do it. Compliance is critical, so experiment a bit and opt for a pattern that works for you. Remember that over time, as you get used to the diet, your body should acclimate to periods of fasting; so keep your personal pattern flexible and adjust to a more lengthy fasting window when you feel able. Stay alert and tweak the regime to suit your needs.

What to Eat

Aim to have food that makes you feel satisfied, but stays firmly within the 500/600-calorie allowance—the best options to achieve this are foods that contain lean protein, and foods with a low Glycemic Index (GI)—for more on this, see page 46. So, stick to the Fast Day mantra: "Mostly Plants and Protein."

The FastDiet does not recommend boycotting carbs entirely, nor does it suggest living permanently on a high-protein diet. We certainly don't advise eating protein to the exclusion of all else on a Fast Day, but you do require an adequate quantity for muscle health, cell maintenance, endocrinal regulation, and immunity. Protein is satiating too, so it's a valuable part of your calorie quota. We recommend that you boost the protein content of your diet on Fast Days, so that it makes up a greater proportion of your diet on just those days. The best advice is to stick to recommended governmental guidelines, which allow for a (quite generous) 50 grams per day. Go for "good protein"—steamed white fish, eggs, shrimp, tofu, and plant protein from nuts, seeds, and legumes (which are also full of fiber and act as bulking agents on a hungry day). When it comes to vegetables, bring in the Double Vs—plenty of Volume, plenty of Variety.

What Does Fasting Feel Like?

If it has been a while since you have experienced hunger, you'll probably find that eating no more than 500 or 600 calories in a day is a mild challenge, at least initially. Intermittent Fasters do report that the process becomes significantly easier with time, particularly as they witness results in the mirror and on the scales. Have faith: your mission is to get through the day.

Getting Past the Lows . . . and Feeling the Highs

There is no reason to be alarmed by benign, occasional, short-term hunger. Given base-level good health, it will do you no harm at all. Your body is designed to go without food for longish periods, even if it has lost the skill through years of routine picking and snacking.

Remember that the diet you may have been used to—a typical Western grazing diet—is almost designed to make you feel hungry, so much so that hunger becomes the white noise of daily life. Try to recognize that what you feel as "hunger" can be a learned reaction to external cues— it's often, as we'll see in chapter 4, "emotional hunger," rather than a true physiological state. There are ways to circumvent the feeling: the real trick is to eat food which keeps you feeling full longer. This means some protein. This means slow-burn, low-GI fuel. This means bulk from plants.

In any case, you're unlikely to be troubled by hunger at all until well into a Fast Day. Fasters also report that the feeling of perceived hunger comes in waves; it will pass. You have absolute power to conquer feelings of hunger simply by steering your mind, riding those waves, choosing to do something else; perhaps drink an herbal tea, go for a walk, get stuck in a sudoku or a movie or a particularly gripping novel. This is an acquired skill, and you'll discover plenty of ways to obtain it in the chapters to come. Some people (Matthew McConaughey among them, apparently) swear that brushing their teeth stops them from feeling hungry . . . Do whatever works for you.

After a few weeks practicing IF, people generally report that their sense of hunger is diminished. So, take heart. On a Fast Day, refrain, restrain, divert, and distract yourself. Before you know it, you've retrained your brain and hunger's off the menu.

One of the reasons that the FastDiet has proved so sustainable for so many is the simple realization that "tomorrow's another day." There's boundless psychological comfort in the fact that your fasting will only be a brief break from food. On the FastBeach Diet, you will still be eating "normally" on non-Fast Days: You'll simply be eating with more awareness than you might on the traditional FastDiet, using techniques to ensure that your food choices are absolutely the best you can make.

Bear in mind, too, that fasters regularly report that the food with which they "break their fast" tastes great; my mother-in-law calls this "hunger sauce"—and if you've never tasted it, you're in for a treat. There's nothing like a bit of delayed gratification to make good things taste even better.

Fast Day Tips

Stay Hydrated

Drink plenty of water. Get into the habit of drinking a glass of water before and after Fast Day meals. And drink water when you feel hungry too (it really does help; the stomach is a simple beast); it will also stop you mistaking thirst for hunger. At the most basic level, drinking water keeps your mouth occupied when it would otherwise be anticipating a snack. Supplement your water intake with herbal tea, black coffee, miso soup—but not juice which, as we'll see on page 57, can rack up the sugars. For more great summertime FastBeach Diet drinks, see pages 61–62.

Axe the Snacks

Remember, your aim is to secure a food-free breathing space for your body. All calories count on a Fast Day, and your objective is to achieve as long a fasting window as possible. Having a complete moratorium on snacking actually makes the process easier to handle: if "no means no," then you avoid questions or calorie calculations. No nibbles, no quibbles. But if you absolutely must snack, make it a good one: have berries, an apple, a carrot. See pages 137–138 for a list of Fast-friendly calorie-counted snacks.

Keep Your Perspective

Going to 510 calories (or 615 for a man) won't hurt—it won't obliterate a fast. But while there's no particular "magic" to 500 or 600 calories, do try to stick broadly to these numbers; you need clear parameters to make the strategy effective in the medium term. And stay positive. Don't be disheartened if you plateau and don't lose weight in any given week; weight loss is your bonus, not your sole objective.

Chapter 4

Introducing the FastDiet Max

As we established in the original *FastDiet* book, in order to be effective, any weight-loss regimen must be sustainable over the long haul. "To work at all," I wrote back then, "any weight-loss strategy has to be tolerable, organic, and innate, not some spurious add-on that makes you feel awkward and self-conscious, the dietary equivalent of uncomfortable shoes . . ." We know that one of the keys to the success of the 5:2 FastDiet is compliance—we do it gladly because the commitment is only occasional and always leavened by the prospect of a day of normal eating tomorrow.

The FastBeach Diet takes a slightly different tack. Think of it as a jump-start. A reboot. It's the turbo-drive button that takes you off cruise control. The idea is to commit to a six-week modified program, knowing that you can soon return to the familiar territory of the classic 5:2. You may want to use it in the run-up to a holiday, a wedding, a moment when you want to shine, a day that demands that you look your best. It's for people who may feel they have got a bit stuck; just as having a dry January or growing a mustache for November has become part of many people's annual calendar, so the FastBeach Diet can be your short-term, souped-up strategy for summer. Its approach is three-pronged, based on ways to:

• Tighten up on Fast Days

• Toughen up on non-Fast Days, and

• Tune in on any day

You may choose to include most of the suggestions here, or just a handful of them. If you want a shorthand checklist of all the FastBeach Diet hints, tips, and techniques, you'll find one at the end of the six-week diet planner included in this book. First, it's time to rev up your Fast Days.

Tighten Up on Fast Days

The simple premise of the FastDiet requires you to cut back hard on calories for two days a week, and it's entirely possible that this is more than enough for you. But on the six-week FastBeach Diet, you should aim to step up the program by experimenting with extensions to the original plan. These are suggestions not imperatives—so read, absorb—and, if it feels right, have a go.

Try 4:3
One clear way to accelerate your FastDiet is to add a third Fast Day each week for six weeks. In practice, this amounts to Alternate Day Fasting (ADF), and is the IF method that

has been most extensively investigated by researchers. To inspire you on your way, consider the following:

• A surprising finding during ADF trials was that people, when allowed to feast on a normal day, did not tend to do so. They reported not feeling particularly hungry after a day of fasting and rarely ate more than 110% of their normal calories.[2]

• Another intriguing finding was that people on this form of IF lost more body fat than those doing a conventional calorie-restricting regimen. If you go on a standard, medically approved diet (i.e., restricting your calorie intake every day) you will lose around 75% of weight as fat, 25% as muscle. On ADF, by contrast, the weight lost is almost entirely fat.

What is also encouraging is that studies done with volunteers who have tried ADF show that those who stick to it report increasing feelings of fullness and dietary satisfaction over time. One explanation for this is that your stomach will shrink. So by all means give ADF or 4:3 a go. If it appeals, try it for six weeks only, always ensuring that you are meeting your nutritional needs over the course of a week—so, plenty of plants, adequate protein, occasional dairy, some "good fats." There's plenty of motivation and support later in this chapter.

Try 2-to-2
Some fasters get quite exercised about the precise timing of a fast. Michael and I are not overly prescriptive on this point:

our aim is to present a flexible plan that can be adapted to suit your own particular lifestyle and daily agenda. That said, it's clear that you can experiment with timing in order to maximize the effectiveness of a fast. You may, for instance, choose to fast, not from bedtime to bedtime, but from 2 p.m. until 2 p.m., with reduced calories (or no calories) consumed at all during that 24-hour period. This is the method proposed by Canadian Brad Pilon in his seminal e-book *Eat Stop Eat* (if you haven't read it, I urge you to, particularly if you are interested in fitness and muscle mass).

If you choose to try the 2-to-2, here's how to go about it: after a normal lunch on Day 1, eat sparingly (or, if you follow Pilon's approach, nothing at all) until a late lunch the following day. That way, you fast as you sleep and no single day feels uncomfortably deprived of food. It's a clever trick, but it does require a modicum more concentration and commitment than the expressly straightforward whole-day option with its 500/600-calorie allowance. You might also choose to fast from dinner to dinner, which again means that no day is All Fast and No Fun. The point is that this plan is "adjust to fit." During the FastBeach Diet, you may want to try a 2-to-2 full 24-hour fast to discover whether it's a good method for you. Stay playful, stay alert. Remember, you are in the driving seat, your foot poised delicately on the gas: if it feels wrong, pull over and revert to your usual 5:2 approach.

Extend Your Fasting Window

Alternatively, you may simply choose to extend your normal fasting window. In the classic FastDiet, we recommend breakfast, perhaps at 7 a.m., then supper around 12 hours later. It's what works for me, and for many women who need a little sustenance to get the day going. This gives us 12 hours without food. However, as we know, plenty of successful FastDieters prefer to ignore breakfast entirely; these people—and I've found them to be mostly men—are effectively fasting for longer: from dinner the previous night to dinner on a Fast Day. On this regime, the fasting window can be as long as 24 hours—as with the 2-to-2. This is something you may decide to try during the FastBeach Diet. Perhaps give it a go for one of your weekly Fast Days. Remember, this is FastDiet Max, and it may not be to everyone's taste or benefit. Keep an open mind, stay strong, but always shut down a fast if it feels overwhelming.

Be Fast-idious About Your Calorie Quota

If you have been on the FastDiet—or indeed, any diet—for a while, it's human instinct to develop a more blasé approach: you feel you know what's what, so you start to slip and an "unconscious non-compliance" creeps in. While 5:2 demands that you "comply" for only two days a week, it is still something of a challenge to apply yourself, to measure and count on those days. It is, as one 5:2 adherent says, "a bit of a chore. And we humans are very good at avoiding chores." For the next six weeks, don't guestimate, don't cheat, don't avoid the chore. Be particular. On Fast Days, renew your vows and be resolute about those calorie quotas. Apps such as MyFitnessPal will help you discover the calorie count of any given food.

Toughen Up on Non-Fast Days

You'll remember that the advice in *The FastDiet* is to "eat well for five days and reduce your calories for two." It's the foundation of the 5:2 approach, but "eating well" remains quite a vague proposition. The general thrust is that you shouldn't dwell upon calorie counting on the five days a week when you're not fasting. But now, on the six-week FastBeach Diet, we're going to toughen up on the non-Fast Days. For a short, contained period, it's time to really eat *well*. This will require some behavioral change, both subtle and direct. Again, you may choose to implement all of the suggestions in the pages ahead, or handpick those that best suit you. The idea here is to make some short-term sacrifices to get yourself beach ready for summer. First up? The tricky subject of booze . . .

Cut Out Alcohol

I've put this first as it is the most effective way I know to kick-start the FastDiet. I'm not expecting you to give up alcohol forever, just for six short weeks. There are fantastically good reasons for doing so—and they're not all about weight loss.

If you're not sure how much good it will do you, a little experiment[3] performed in the offices of the *New Scientist* may be enough to get you on the wagon. On October 5, 2013, 14 members of the magazine's staff—all of whom considered themselves to be "normal" drinkers—were given a range of tests to gauge the state of their livers and overall health. For the next five weeks, 10 of them drank no alcohol, while the other four continued as normal. Just over a month later, they returned to repeat the tests. For the four drinkers, there had been no significant changes. But in the abstainers, the impact had been dramatic. Their levels of liver fat—a precursor to liver damage—had fallen by an average of 15%. Their blood glucose levels had fallen a staggering 23% from 5.1 to 4.3mmol/l (the normal range is 3.9–5.6). They'd lost weight—3.5 pounds on average. And their total blood cholesterol, a risk factor for heart disease, had dropped on average by 5%, from 4.6 to 4.4 mmo/l (a healthy level is anything below 5.2 mmo/l). The abstainers also reported sleeping better (up to 10% on the scale), and having improved concentration.

As the *New Scientist* went on to report in its January 2014 issue, Kevin Moore, a consultant in liver services at University College London Medical School, declared himself amazed by the results. "What you have is a pretty average group of people who would not consider themselves heavy drinkers, yet stopping drinking *for a month* [my italics] alters liver fat, cholesterol, and blood sugar and helps them lose weight. If someone did that with a health product, they'd be raking it in."

If that's not quite enough to convince you, here are five more very good reasons to decline the wine for a brief period in order to jump-start your FastDiet:

• Alcohol is chemically similar to sugar, so drinking it will set off the same insulin resistance that can promote weight gain.

• It is loaded with calories and largely devoid of any nutritional benefit. A recent survey found that 85% of consumers don't know how many calories are in a glass of wine, and 63% don't consider wine when counting their calorie intake.[4] But an 8-ounce glass of wine contains around 180 calories, a similar number to ice cream; and remember—the higher the alcohol content, the more calories you're getting (see box below).

• Alcohol inhibits sleep (find out why this isn't great for weight loss on pages 62–64).

• It also stimulates appetite.

• Nutritionists recognize that the body processes alcohol before it gets to work on fats and carbs—which means that drinking slows down the burning of fat for energy.

In short, if you're really serious about trying to lose weight and gain health, consider a complete ban on alcohol for the duration of your FastBeach Diet. You can always tuck into the sangria once you're on vacation.

CAN'T REJECT? THEN REDUCE

If you simply want to drink in a more controlled way during your six-week FastBeach Diet, a few subtle changes can really cut your calorie count:
• Only fill your glass halfway.
• Make every second drink water.

- Keep the opened wine bottle in the fridge or cupboard, not on the table, where it's easier to reach for a refill.
- Swap white wine for spritzers.
- Keep adding ice cubes.
- Choose small glasses (a "glass of wine" used to be one unit; now—thanks to more generous glass sizes—it's two). And do be aware of visual illusions: research shows that people pour 28% more into short, wide glasses than tall ones.[5]
- Watch your mixers. Soda water, lemon, and lime juice are the best bet; orange juice will double the calorie count of a vodka shot.
- Choose at least one night a week when you give alcohol a pass.

THE CALORIES IN YOUR GLASS

Alcohol has around seven calories per gram, nearly twice that of protein or carbs, and is almost as calorific as fat. Brands and serving sizes will differ, but the following list gives a rough idea of the average calories in your drink.

Drink	Serving size	Calories
Bitter	1 pint	180
Lager	1 pint	150–240

Champagne	1 glass (4 ounces)	90
White wine	1 glass (4 ounces)	85
Red wine	1 glass (4 ounces)	80
Shot of gin	1 ounce	55
Shot of vodka	1 ounce	55
Whisky	1 ounce	55
Rum & Diet Coke	9 ounces	55
Glass of Baileys	1.3 ounces	120
Red Bull	8 ounces	110
Orange juice	8 ounces	115
Lemon juice	1 tablespoon	4
Lime juice	1 tablespoon	4

Shift Your Eating on Non-Fast Days

So, for six weeks only, you'll need to watch what you eat on non-Fast Days as well as Fast Days and exert a degree of dietary restraint; the good news is that even modest changes in the way that you eat and the way that you think can really make a difference.

Here's your best bet for success on the FastBeach Diet:

• On a Fast Day, follow the 500/600-calorie rule.

• On a non-Fast Day, eat healthily, moderately, and with awareness.

Simple, yes. But what does it mean in practice? On the FastBeach Diet you do need to rethink a few attitudes, actions, and habits in order to fulfil the "eat healthily" part of the bargain. It's not a revolution. It's a recalibration, a time to reset your habits and expectations around food. Without assiduous calorie counting, it's now worth holding back on indulgences—the empty calories, extra helpings, and superfluous snacks which may usually be part of your non-Fast Days.

The following are suggestions, not edicts, a host of ideas for you to try, like a buffet of ways to introduce healthy eating into your life. Some may seem obvious, some you'll be doing already, others may steer you on a new course. The idea is to introduce as many healthy habits as possible over the course of your FastBeach Diet, exercising just a bit more informed caution, a little more vigilance. So, pick and mix, remembering to keep it fairly simple and not so restrictive as to impact harshly upon your everyday life. This is not meant to be a punishment, and you shouldn't become a martyr to the cause. Here's how to accomplish the shift, realistically, positively, and wisely.

Be Far Less Refined

"People who eat white bread have no dreams!" proclaimed the great fashion editor Diana Vreeland—and, for some reason, her call to unrefined carbs has always stuck in my mind. One vital shift in thinking for FastBeach Diet purposes is to recognize the difference between fast-acting and slow-acting carbohydrates.

For the next six weeks, focus on low-GI carbs which are slow burning (oatmeal, brown basmati rice, stone-ground whole grain bread) rather than fast burning (cake, crumpets, white bread). This is your best bet to bypass the sugar cycle—the familiar crave, consume, crash, crave, consume, crash spiral that we're keen to avoid during the FastBeach Diet.

WHY INSULIN MATTERS

Highly refined carbs have a high Glycemic Index (GI) and cause a spike in your blood sugar levels, which then leads your pancreas to produce insulin. Insulin reduces the level of glucose in the bloodstream by diverting it to various body tissues for immediate use—or by storing it as fat. It also inhibits the conversion of body fat back into glucose for the body to burn. So insulin both facilitates the accumulation of fat, and then guards against its depletion. Insulin also acts on the brain to make you eat more, on your liver to manufacture more fat, and on the fat cells in your belly to store that fat. A steady blood sugar level—encouraged by those slow-burn carbs which take time and energy to digest—will elicit a lower insulin response that can help to regulate your appetite. In other words, you're less likely to feel as hungry.

GETTING TO GRIPS WITH GI, GL, AND IL

While I'd always recommend that you don't over-think these things, it's worth having an eye on the blood-sugar impact of the foods you eat during your FastBeach Diet.

As accustomed dieters will know, one way to discover which carbs cause a spike and which don't is to look at their Glycemic Index (GI). Each food gets a score out of a 100 (pure sugar scores 100 on the GI scale). A low score means that the particular food does not tend to cause a rapid rise in blood glucose. These are the ones you want.

Of course, the size of the sugar spike depends not just on the food itself, but also on how much of it you eat. So there's also a measure called the Glycemic Load (GL):

$$\frac{\text{GI x grams of carbohydrate}}{100}$$

You can find GI and GL scores for most carbs online. Do recognize that the numbers can be somewhat arbitrary and occasionally contradictory—so if you want to have precise numbers, perhaps take an average of several sources. The American Diabetes Association has an excellent guide at www.diabetes.org.

More recently, nutritionists have started to turn their attention to the Insulin Load (IL) based on a given food's Insulin Index[6]—a number designed to reveal which foods give a surge of insulin by measuring the postprandial increase in insulin secretion of a whole food, including the interactions between, say, carbs, proteins, and fats. This is the crunch. What you really want to know on your FastBeach Diet is which foods are likely to promote a lower insulin response than others. Oatmeal, for example, elicits a lower insulin response than muesli; milk has a higher than expected IL, as does beef. As a general rule of thumb, foods with a high Insulin Index include refined cereals, sweets, white bread, and potatoes, while most vegetables—no surprise here—produce a negligible insulin response.

Cook at Home

Three easy little words. But quite a tricky concept to work into everyday life if you're up to your neck in work and kids, and the frozen meal is right there, looking so very convenient in its plastic jacket and jazzy sleeve. I understand. Cooking from scratch doesn't always fit. But try to make time to cook, just for the next six weeks. If you can't do it daily, do it often. If you can't do it often, do it sometimes (in batches, then freeze it).

You may, of course, already be a kitchen connoisseur: now it's time to get those calorie counts down. Remember, home cooking means you can control the quality and the quantity of what you eat; besides, cooking in summertime really is a breeze—sometimes a simple question of opening the crisper drawer and grabbing the cutting board (do ensure that your fridge can deliver; see pages 140–141 for a quick Fast-friendly shopping list). Check out chapter 7 for plenty of FastDiet cooking tips and my new summer recipes—many of which take less time to prepare than it takes to unwrap a frozen meal and get it to go ping—or look at the hundreds of ideas in *The FastDiet Recipe Book* and *FastCook*.

Cut Back on Treats

"Treats." Remember those? An occasional pleasure. A rare delight. I don't want to get all misty-eyed and rose-tinted, but when I was a child, a treat was exactly that: a piece of fudge, a custard cream, two lemon sherbets, something you had sometimes, not always, when you'd been particularly good. These days, "treats" are almost a food group in their own right. You only have to get in line to pay at a gas station to be engulfed in a roiling sea of snacks and grab bags and cookies and chocolate and STOP! Let's get some perspective here and put the treats back in their box. Not forever. Just for a bit.

One of the pillars of the success of the FastDiet is, of course, that it expressly allows occasional treats: it's what makes the program sustainable and feasible over the long term. Hallelujah. But during the FastBeach Diet, it's time for tough love. Rather than eliminate, recalibrate. Remember, it's ONLY FOR SIX WEEKS (did I mention that?).

Packaging? Pack It In

One super-simple way to facilitate healthy eating is to gravitate toward foods with very little packaging: the ratio of plastic to food is generally a pretty good indication of its nutritional value. Products that don't require much in the way of packaging tend to feature fewer stabilizers and additives than their overly packaged cousins.

While following the FastBeach Diet, also beware of "low-fat" foods, where the fat has often simply been replaced with sugar. They have a "health halo" effect that can actually encourage you to eat more (curiously, research has shown that low-fat labels lead people to eat 16–23% more calories in total)[7]. Similarly, don't fall for the seductive health claims on the packet. Words like "wholesome" are largely puff, designed to make you feel good and fish out your wallet. Better to read the back of the package than the front.

Ban the Big No-Nos

The list of foods to avoid throughout the FastBeach Diet will come as no surprise: packaged desserts, sweet fizzy drinks, commercial cereals, and fast food should all be out of bounds for the next month and a half. But there's one killer combo that you really need to eliminate for as long as possible . . .

CUT THE 50:50S

Foods high in fat or sugar, as we all know, can be very appealing, but what has recently been discovered is that in combination they are *particularly* tempting; we crave this mix and we find it very difficult to stop eating it once we've got going. According to neuroscientist

Professor Paul Kenny at the Scripps Research Institute in Florida, food with a 50:50 fat:sugar ratio interferes with our mechanisms of self-regulation;[8] there's simply no off switch, as there would be when consuming either macronutrient alone. Scientists call this "hedonic eating." It supercharges the brain's reward system and overrides satiety signals. Interestingly, this particular 50:50 fat sugar ratio doesn't happen in nature. But it does happen in cheesecake. And doughnuts. And those moist chocolate fudge cakes that look so fetching in supermarkets and coffee shops, the saucy sirens of the bakery world. So, make a commitment. No 50:50s for the duration of the FastBeach Diet. None. I bet they'll look a lot less alluring after six weeks . . .

Go Mediterranean

One way to ensure that you eat healthily and wisely throughout your FastBeach Diet is to stick to a Mediterranean diet on the five days a week when you're not fasting. "Mediterranean" is a shorthand way of saying "cut the junk and get real." This approach will be familiar to anyone who has read Dr. Michelle Harvie's *2-Day Diet*, based on her research at the Genesis Breast Cancer Prevention Centre. The idea is to follow a carefully defined and controlled diet for two consecutive days, and then stick to fruit, vegetables, whole grains, beans, legumes, nuts, olive oil, lean protein, and unsweetened dairy on your five "non-diet" days each week.

It is certainly an effective way to lose weight. In her studies Dr. Harvie found that female dieters who stuck to her plan for 12 weeks lost an average of 14 pounds and 2 inches from their waists and hips. Some did much better, losing as much as 32 pounds and dropping two dress sizes. So a six-week sabbatical in the Mediterranean? Why not?

Think Summer, Eat Summer

Another way to sharpen up your eating habits at this time of year is simply, consciously, to embrace the season. As the days lengthen and the weather improves, it's easier—in fact, it's obvious—to shift to fewer carbs and fats, more salads and fresh veggies. Here's how to go about it:

- **Change how you cook to suit summer:** simply going from fried to grilled and using a multilevel steamer will save significant calories on any day of the week.

- **Roll out the barbecue:** it's one of the best low-cal ways to cook protein, whether it's slapped direct on the grill or wrapped in foil and tucked into the embers.

- **Go raw:** the idea—if you want to stick to the method advocated by "raw foodists"—is that nothing should be heated beyond 244°F (the point at which some vitamins are lost). During your FastBeach Diet, consider introducing a raw day once a week (on a Fast or a non-Fast Day). It's worth noting that some nutrients are less available in raw foods than cooked—the beta carotene in carrots, for example, or the lycopene in tomatoes. But a raw day is a great way to treat yourself to fresh tastes and a fresh approach, shaking up old eating habits. Try Pen's beet salad on page 131 for inspiration. Or—a startlingly simple suggestion—just eat more Japanese food. The Japanese have some of the lowest obesity rates in the developed world, in part because their diet contains a lot of food served in varying degrees of rawness.

• **Go fish:** the Japanese also tend to consume a good deal less meat than Westerners. Fish are high in protein and some, such as salmon, mackerel, and tuna—the oily fish—are also high in omega-3 essential fatty acids (though higher in calories too). Go for sashimi over sushi (that way, you avoid rice) for the perfect summer dinner. For an Italian version of sashimi, try crudo: slice ultra-fresh raw fish—bass, flounder, or mackerel—into tissue-thin strips and serve with a little olive oil, lemon, and fresh herbs rather than the usual trio of Japanese accompaniments.

A SIMPLE SUMMER CEVICHE

If you find completely raw fish a challenge, try ceviche, where acid in a citrus marinade "cooks" the fish without heat. This is a traditional Latin American method—which also happens to be deeply fashionable at the moment (perhaps as a response to our newly acquired taste for low-carb food). Not surprisingly, it requires the freshest fish you can find.

Combine the juice of a lime and the juice of a lemon with one finely diced red onion, one red chili pepper (seeded and finely chopped, to taste), salt and pepper, and a dash of Tabasco. Add a good handful of chopped cilantro and a fillet of fresh fish, boned, skinned, and cubed or sliced, per person. Place all the ingredients in a nonreactive bowl and refrigerate for half an hour, then serve.

Have Soup Before Dinner . . . or at Any Time

Soup, according to research from Penn State University,[9] is a great appetite suppressant because it consists of a hunger-busting combination of liquids and solids; eat it before a meal and you can lower your overall calorie intake by up to 20% compared to a meal without soup. So eat soup—winter warm or summer chilled—regularly during your six-week FastBeach Diet. A light veggie broth is an ideal way to get water and fiber into your stomach to start to signal fullness before you embark on the meal proper.

On a non-Fast Day, consider replacing your usual lunch-time sandwich with a simple soup—just doing this will eliminate 10 slices of bread (and butter) from your weekly consumption. To keep the calories under control, choose vegetable-based broths rather than thick creamy or meaty soups, the kind you can stand your spoon up in. Me? I'm a sucker for pho, a Vietnamese broth packed with fresh herbs and chili peppers. Look out for it on your lunchtime takeout menu, or make your own, following the recipe on pages 134–135.

Implement the Rule of Three-Quarters

You want simple? Here's simple. Fill your plate with vegetables at the expense of meat and carbs—a 75:25 ratio would be ideal. This single, relatively small change can make a huge difference to your calorie and nutrient intake over the course of the six weeks.

It's no surprise to learn that we in the rich world eat three or four times as much animal protein as we need, and most of the nutrients we get from our meat mania are just as available from plants (5 ounces of nuts and seeds a day will do the job).

While meat is generally a good source of protein and certain micronutrients, it can be high in saturated fat and cholesterol. Studies have found that a vegan or vegetarian diet can be highly effective for weight loss,[10] and vegetarian populations tend to have lower rates of heart disease, high blood pressure, diabetes, and obesity.[11]

Even if wholesale vegetarianism isn't on your agenda, cutting back on red and processed meat consumption certainly makes sense on any number of levels—at least for the duration of your FastBeach Diet. So how else can you start the shift?

• Institute a meat-free day each week—a Meatless Monday, perhaps. Or go further and stay meat free all week, with meat reserved for a weekend treat.

• Avoid the "meat as main course" mentality; think veggies first. Give plants a starring role on your plate, not a bit part.

• Cook plants as you would meat—roast, grill, broil, bake—
to give them that central function.

There's another, perhaps more pedestrian, advantage to
increasing the vegetable content of your meals, and it has
to do with bulk. Eating "big" foods containing plenty of
fiber and water—loads of leaves, stacks of salad, great piles
of greens—will fill you up for fewer calories. That's what
you want in the weeks ahead.

A QUICK WORD ON VITAMIN C

Fiber. Nutrients. Volume. Yes, you already know
eating plenty of vegetables makes sense. What you
may not know is that vitamin C, among its many
health benefits, may well be crucial for weight
management. According to researchers from
Arizona State University, individuals who consume
an adequate amount of vitamin C burn 30% more
fat during moderate exercise than those who don't
get enough of the stuff.[12] They also showed that
too little vitamin C in the bloodstream correlates
with increased body fat and waist measurements.
Remember that vitamin C is easily lost—so if you're
cooking leafy veggies, do it quickly. Steaming is
ideal.

Watch What You Drink

We've already talked about limiting your alcohol intake while on the FastBeach Diet; but there are equally good reasons for cutting back on soft drinks too. While many of us are aware of the calories loaded on our forks, the ones that lurk in cups and glasses frequently go uncounted. You may well need to modify your behavior, so make the commitment, write it down, and have alternatives at hand. As you'll discover later in this chapter, with recognition and repetition, habits can be modified. After six weeks, your daily caramel latte will seem about as appealing as a triple-layer cream cake with cream on the side.

First, Junk the Juice

Beware the "health halo" of smoothies and juices. Fruit juice is ultimately a higher-sugar, lower-fiber version of its source. Juicing eliminates the skins of the fruits, precisely where most of their health-giving flavonoids and carotenoids are concentrated; the skins are also the primary source of fiber— important for the health of your gut, and useful in slowing down the digestion and absorption of the juice's sugars.

Commercial smoothies can have a similar sugar content to soda and, because they are acidic, they are corrosive to your teeth; they are also loaded with calories. Have an apple instead, or choose one of the drinks in the Fast-friendly list on pages 61–62.

If you are thinking about trying vegetable juices as an alternative, be aware that carrot and tomato juice are at the higher end of the calorie spectrum, while green vegetable juice is at the lower end.

THE GREEN GREEN JUICE OF HOME

Trendy? Yes. Faddish? Possibly. But green juices do have substantial nutritional value, and significantly less sugar than their fruit equivalents. They usually involve great gusts of leafy vegetables and brassicas such as kale, spinach, chard, or broccoli—far more than you could possibly consume in a single sitting. The dark green vegetables contain a glorious cargo of vitamins and minerals—so it's little wonder that many fasters swear by them to start the day, and all for wonderfully few calories. You may like to try some of these favorite combinations:

- Kale, mint, and apple
- Spinach, green greens, Tuscan kale, apple, and lemon juice
- Watercress, parsley, cucumber, and ginger
- Romaine lettuce, celery, and green pear
- Arugula, spinach, pear, and lime

But a few rules of thumb:

- Don't store it; drink green juice immediately as it degrades quickly.
- You'll be getting the vitamins and minerals of your chosen vegetables, but far less of their soluble fiber—which is the really good stuff for your cholesterol and blood pressure.
- Your best bet is a fresh green juice rather than a bottled one, which will almost certainly have been

pasteurized—great for its shelf life, but not for its nutritional value.
- Be careful with green juices if you are on anti-depressants or blood-thinning meds.

No Soda . . . Sorry, Not Even Diet Coke

Most fasters will have already eliminated "full-fat" fizzy drinks from their repertoire on a Fast Day, knowing that they're liquid calorie traps. Good reasons, then, to drop the pop for the duration of the FastBeach Diet on non-Fast Days too. You can do it. We can help. Look at the list below for dozens of no-cal and low-cal drinks, with a particular emphasis on delicious and unusual summertime tastes.

But what about the tricky question of diet soda? I know that lots of FastDiet fans rely on a Diet Coke to get them through to dinner with their temper intact. But, listen up: counterintuitive as it may seem, some studies suggest that consuming zero-calorie sweeteners *increases* the risk of putting on weight.[13] Scientists at Purdue University in Indiana analyzed the link and found that rats fed yogurt sweetened with saccharin (a sugar substitute) ate more, and grew fatter, than those eating yogurt sweetened with glucose (the real thing). The researchers submitted that sweet foods provide an "orosensory stimulus" that convinces the body that a deluge of calories is on its way. When, as with diet drinks, the advertised calories don't materialize, the system becomes confused—and as a result "people eat more or expend less energy than they otherwise would."

Even if you're not convinced by this line of reasoning, what's indisputable is that the makers of processed diet foods and drinks tend to replace fats and sugars with synthetic alternatives and "lab-designed" compounds. During the FastBeach Diet, try to wean yourself off the fake foods like these. Again, habit can be a surprisingly fragile beast: fight it for a while and it will almost certainly disappear, like a shadow when you turn on the light.

Choose Your Coffee Carefully

There's a growing body of evidence to suggest that, far from being a guilty pleasure, coffee may be good for you, helping to prevent mental decline, improve cardiac health, and reduce the risk of diabetes, liver cancer, and stroke.[14] It does matter, however, what you order from your friendly local barista. A Starbucks grande whole-milk caffé mocha with whipped cream, to take one ridiculous example, has 396 calories. Even a caffé latte with skim milk has 71. And a double espresso? Just 11. So, decide right now to ditch the gaudy coffees that have danced into our lives and taken up lazy residence. Try instead, just for this six weeks, to drink your coffee black and sugarless. If you still despise it after several attempts, have just a dash of milk to take the edge off. Remember: the FastBeach Diet is a short, sharp wake-up call, and for the next six weeks you do need to stay gently alert, like a seated (not sleeping) guard at the gate.

WHAT TO DRINK IN SUMMERTIME

- Vanilla tea—hot or chilled. Add a slice or two of fresh ginger root.
- Coconut water—a good alternative to sports drinks, it's natural and low in sugar (it still has 83 calories per 11 ounces, though, so go easy).
- If tap water doesn't turn you on, buy a water filter and keep a jug of filtered water in the fridge, perhaps with added slices of lemon, lime, mint, lemongrass, basil leaves, or cucumber.
- Chilled herbal tea—try peppermint tea over ice with crushed fresh mint leaves. Iced cranberry and pomegranate tea are great too—keep them in the fridge and serve with slices of fresh orange.
- Hot water with lemon and ginger; or with cloves, lemongrass, or even a slice of red chili peppers.
- Green tea—plenty of people believe in the fat-busting, antioxidant power of green tea. But all you really need to absorb is that it has virtually no calories, and about half the caffeine of coffee.
- The same goes for Chinese pu-er tea, which comes in cake form, to be crumbled into boiling water. Devotees speak of its capacity to reduce cholesterol and raise the metabolic rate; again, the jury's out—but if you enjoy it, dive right in.
- Virgin mojito, made with soda, mint, lime, and

a bruised lemongrass stalk to stir. Serve on the rocks in a tall glass.

- Homemade lemon iced tea—make a tea of your choice (English breakfast can't be beaten), chill, add lemon or orange slices, or a squeeze of juice and thin tendrils of the zest. Add a teaspoon of agave if you need a little sweetener.
- No-added sugar cordials diluted with still or sparkling water. Freeze diluted elderflower cordials into popsicles or ice cubes to have on hot days.
- Iced black coffee—simply pour espresso over ice cubes and sip.
- At bedtime, if sleep is elusive, try warm skim milk with nutmeg, a dash of vanilla extract, and a cinnamon stick to stir.

Sleep Well

There are dozens of published research papers that link poor sleep with weight gain. Researchers at the University of Warwick analyzed the relationship between sleep and obesity and found that adults who slept for fewer than five hours a night were one and a half times more likely to be obese.[15] Why?

The answer comes from studies of leptin and ghrelin, two of the hormones that govern appetite. For some reason, I think of them as characters from *The Lord of the Rings*—leptin, the elf that keeps the hypothalamus informed about the adequacy of your energy stores, is the satiety hormone that suppresses appetite; ghrelin is the belly dwarf whose job it is to signal hunger to the brain.

Leptin, secreted by fat cells, has a circadian rhythm and reaches its peak during sleep. If you're not sleeping well, peak leptin levels are not reached and the brain sends out its minions—hunger pangs and energy conservation. At the same time, lack of sleep causes ghrelin levels to rise. Your appetite kicks in and calorie-dense, dopamine-generating snacks become irresistible.

There have been innumerable investigations—sometimes resulting in hyperbolic claims—into sleep and its effect on leptin and ghrelin. A swift roundup might include:

• A study of 1,000 volunteers at Stanford University found that those who slept fewer than eight hours a night had lower levels of leptin and higher levels of ghrelin, and they also had higher levels of body fat. "Specifically, those who slept the fewest hours per night weighed the most."[16]

• Researchers at Bristol University compared blood samples from insomniacs and good sleepers.[17] The former had leptin levels 15% below normal, and ghrelin levels 15% above normal.

• A study at Laval University in Quebec found that there may be an ideal "sleep zone" of around eight hours a night that facilitates body-weight regulation.[18]

None of this is incontrovertible evidence that a good night's sleep will encourage fat loss on your FastBeach Diet. But it is worth knowing that sleep is far from a passive state; disrupt it and our bodies will inevitably suffer. Besides, whatever our hormones are doing, poor sleep will certainly rob us of the energy required to bounce out of bed and make the best of a day. This low-energy cycle is the enemy of sustainable weight loss, since sugary, salty, starchy snacks are incomparably more enticing when we're tired.

So, commit to going to bed at a reasonable time while on your diet. Try and get a decent eight-hour sleep every night for the next six weeks (much easier, incidentally, when you go alcohol free). It will do you a world of good, and may even help shift those scales.

HOW TO GET YOUR ZZZZS WITH EASE

- Institute a screen ban: no screens, no tablets, no phones at bedtime. If your bedroom looks like the control room at NASA, unplug it now.
- Get up at a regular time: no matter when you went to sleep, rise at the same time each day. This helps to program your body clock into a good sleep–wake pattern, which can be hugely helpful for insomniacs.
- Nap with care: if you're feeling done in by mid-afternoon, take just a short 15-minute nap. Beyond that, you'll eat into your body's sleep needs and may disrupt your night.

Tune In on Any Day

You'll have already absorbed that 5:2 is a limited but effective discipline; what it requires is a change of behavior. A change of mind. Part of its intention (and one of the prime reasons for its success) is that it encourages you to be observant, "mindful," around food—certainly on your two Fast Days. On the FastBeach Diet, you need to be that much more aware, for that much more of the time. This needn't be a burden; it can be a fascinating undertaking that serves to illuminate entrenched behavior around food and eating.

In addition, it's important to get a handle on habit, on temptation, and on cravings—the trio of trips that can up-end you on the fast track to weight loss and good health. It's time to retrain your brain.

Cultivate Mindfulness Around Food

Mindfulness is a fashionable concept these days, but it is rooted in age-old wisdom that can, and should, affect your relationship with everything in your world, including calories. The key is to live consciously. I'm keen on a quote from Henry Miller, who said that "the aim of life is to live, and to live means to be aware, joyously, drunkenly, serenely, divinely aware." Sounds gorgeous, right? But what does it mean in practice, particularly with regard to the food on your plate? Here are my tips for mindful eating:

- **Don't eat on auto-pilot**. Throughout the diet, eat with awareness, allowing yourself to absorb the fascinating fact that you're eating. Don't eat on the way to doing something else. Don't read, watch TV, text, Facebook, drive, or juggle at the same time. Tune in to the food on your fork. Look at it. Really taste it. That way, you'll enjoy each mouthful. You'll also know when you've had enough. On non-Fast Days, stay alert. Eat until you're satisfied, not until you're full (this will come naturally after a few weeks' practice).

• **Slow down**. It seems a simple enough suggestion, but just think about how often you scarf down your food. For the duration of your FastBeach Diet, sit to eat. Stay put in one place. Make it an event. Eat at a table. Drink a glass of water first. Say grace, if that's your thing. Anything to make you tune in. Eat with intent. Put down your knife and fork between bites. Let your body know what's just hit it, recognizing that it takes your stomach a few minutes to catch up with your mouth; wait 10 minutes before that extra spoonful. Wait again before embarking on dessert. You may not need it today.

• **Guard against portion distortion**. This is the thinking that convinces us that the food piled on our plates—or the amount that is given to us in a "serving"—is the quantity we really want and need. It's a habit, nothing more. So break it. Learn when to say "when." Have a care for the amount of food you're putting on your plate at every meal. Bear in mind that a person will eat an average of 92% of any food they serve themselves.[19] So, for the next six weeks, serve a bit less.

Be particularly aware when ordering food when you're out. Portion sizes have rocketed over the last 20 years—compare a modern cupcake to the cupcakes of your childhood—thanks in part to the availability of cheap food and the marketing practices of the food industry. But we humans are prone to a behavior that psychologists call "unit bias": if the food is moderately palatable, we'll go on eating the amount that's put in front of us until it's gone; we also tend to eat more when offered more.[20] Once you absorb this, you'll realize you really can put the brakes on.

- **Give yourself visual clues**. Yes, smaller plates can be a startlingly effective way to limit your eating (studies have shown that moving from a 12-inch to a 10-inch dinner plate leads people to serve and eat 22% less);[21] dark plates are also thought to be helpful, since you can more clearly discern the amount of food in front of you.

- **Wait before you eat**. Don't eat as soon as the clock says "lunchtime." If you feel hungry during a Fast Day—or on a non-Fast Day during the next six weeks—try to resist for at least 10 minutes to see whether the hunger subsides (as it naturally tends to do). The idea is to put food in its place. It's only food. Once you start to think about food in a rational and realistic way, you'll discover that you can modify your behavior around it. You can even playfully push it aside. You may discover, as many fasters attest, that you develop a keen sensitivity to your own appetite, hunger, and satiety. These will change from day to day. Stay quiet, and you can begin to feel these subtle, visceral things. In time—and six weeks is enough time—you'll learn to turn the dial this way or that, up or down, depending on your needs on any given day.

- **Keep a food diary**. Dieters who keep food diaries are known to be more successful at losing weight than those who don't, with one study finding that it can double weight loss as part of a managed program.[22] Logging one's consumption seems to heighten awareness; the simple act of quantifying incoming food (and, don't forget, drink) seems to be enough to still your hand as it wanders toward the cookies. During the FastBeach Diet, catalog your intake on Fast Days and non-Fast Days, using the planner included in this book.

Temptation, Habit, and Cravings: How to Negotiate the Hurdles Ahead

On average, we make 227 food-related decisions every day (most people, when questioned, wildly underestimate the number and guess that it's about 14).[23] That's plenty of choice, and plenty of opportunities to fall facedown into the nearest pie.

On a diet, most of us are subject to what social psychologists call "dynamic inconsistency"—we tumble into the gap between what we plan in good faith and what we do in real time. And what usually gets in the way or leads us astray is a potent cocktail of temptation, habit, and the collapse of willpower in the face of cravings.

Tackling Temptation

Your mission for the next six weeks, and perhaps beyond, is to recognize temptation for what it is. Temporal. Transient. Fleeting and ephemeral. It is also particular to you. While there are universal experiences, temptation—like love and death—is intensely personal; your job is to unravel what makes you succumb, then try and avert and subvert it. And there are plenty of acknowledged ways to do this:

• **Act upon the Proximity Principle** and put temptation out of reach. One study (using Hershey's Kisses) showed how having food conveniently close makes you eat a great deal more of it.[24] When workers kept the chocolate on their desk, they ate an average of nine Kisses per day; when it was moved just six feet away, they ate only four per day. So, for the next six weeks, remove temptation. Don't give yourself the choice of whether to eat the potato chips or not; don't put the potato chips on the table. Better yet, don't buy them.

• **Conversely, make healthy food abundantly available.** Have it at hand. At mealtimes, serve vegetables and salads in help-yourself bowls on the dining table—but serve meat, cheese, bread, pasta, potatoes, and dessert away from the table to prevent the idle digging-in of a finger or a fork.

• **Just cook enough.** Not too much, but just enough, remembering that leftovers are somehow all the more delicious for being left over.

• **For the next six weeks, don't eat straight from a box**, bag, carton, or tub. Serve yourself a bowl of—whatever—and then put the carton away. Research has also shown that people eat more when given a larger container of food than when they're given a smaller container.[25] So think petite.

• **Don't get sidetracked.** It's worth noting that if you are distracted, you are more likely to give into temptation; in one study, students trying to remember a telephone number were 50% more likely to choose chocolate cake over fruit from a snack cart.[26] When your mind is preoccupied, it makes impulsive, "primitive brain" choices based on urges and instincts; this sits nicely with our ideas about mindful eating. Your job is to tune in and choose right.

- **Your goal must outweigh your temptation.** This may seem obvious (otherwise, you'd never get going). But you need reminding, at the very instant that your hand gravitates toward the bread and the butter. So try site-specific aversion therapy. If necessary, tape a picture of yourself—the selfie you'd never post on Facebook, the holiday snap that made you embark on the FastDiet in the first place—to the fridge door. Simple and aggressive, but effective.

Habits: How to Make Them, How to Break Them

Our mission on the FastBeach Diet is to find ways to happily abstain in a world of incomparable abundance. As Aristotle said, "We are what we repeatedly do"; it's time now to dismantle poor habits and install the good. Popular thinking has it (probably erroneously) that it takes just 21 days to make or break a habit—the truth, however, is that the timing depends largely on what that habit is, and who's doing it. One study at University College London found that it took 66 days to adopt the habit of eating fruit daily, while the habit of drinking a glass of water after breakfast took just 20 days to install.[27] The important thing is to repeat, and repeat, and repeat. As the study (and Aristotle) said, "With repetition of a behavior in a consistent context, automaticity increases." That's what you want. This is subtle stuff—a call to rewire your brain. Here's how to go about it:

• **Change the record.** A study has revealed that up to 45% of what we do every day is habitual[28]—performed without thinking in the same place at the same time in the same bovine way. We respond, automatically, to outside stimuli. Acting without thinking is a central driver of habits. Think about checking your emails. Getting a coffee. Where you sit to watch TV. The route you take on your bike to work. "Habits are formed when the memory associates specific actions with specific places or moods," Professor Wendy Wood of Duke University in North Carolina told the *New York Times*, "If you regularly eat chips while sitting on the couch, after a while, seeing the couch will automatically prompt you to reach for the Doritos."

Your mission for the next six weeks is to undermine your instinctive bias for the status quo. Turn left when you usually turn right. Sit on a different seat on the subway. Take the stairs, not the elevator. When you experience a compulsion to eat too much, or to eat badly, it's time to face it head on. You are a rational being and you are making a specific, time-sensitive decision to eat that cheeseburger or pour that glass of wine. You really do have the power to choose, at each incremental, individual moment. Once you recognize this power, it is possible to overcome the cognitive bias that leads to impulsive snacking and compulsive eating. Try to install a behavior—not forever, just for this precise moment—which alters your established route. This is called "deliberate practice"; it takes grit and determination. Leave the table. Stretch your legs. Don't eat in front of the TV (throw out the tray that makes it possible). Change the picture.

- **Be specific**. Research shows that vague plans are more likely to fail—so avoid abstraction, waffling, and generalizations. Think through exactly what you are going to do, where you are going to do it, and at what time. For example, instead of saying that you will go running two days a week, tell yourself that you will run on Sundays and Wednesdays at 7 p.m. Instead of saying "I'll cut back on treats" say "I won't have my morning muffin." Similarly, as we've established above, if you want to lose weight, there is a psychological advantage in setting a specific goal for how much weight (10 pounds?), by when (August 15 when you fly to Miami?).

- **Think carrots, not sticks**. A study from the University of Chicago outlines how positive feedback on new habits will increase the likelihood of success.[29] Don't be afraid to recognize and grandstand your achievements. Website forums make an ideal platform for a bit of back patting—go to www.thefastdiet.co.uk to find tons of support and praise in action. Plenty of people on our site say that this is often enough to get them through a tricky patch.

- **Decode your brain**. Appetite is governed by a complex interaction of hormones, neurotransmitters, and enzymes—and we don't have a clear picture of the precise interrelations at work as we eat, or as we fast. What we do know is that hunger has a biochemical basis: grasping just a little about what your hormones are up to can really help when you're attempting to change habits or overcome temptation. Let's return to leptin, the satiety hormone which encourages you to stop eating when you're full. Its message can be readily overcome by the reward systems in your brain.[30] This "hedonic eating" may be a response to any number of outside influences: you'll recognize it if you eat for reasons other than hunger. The kicker might be social (shared lunches, communal eating, everyone at the table agreeing to order dessert); it may be environmental (scheduled mealtimes which persuade you that you're hungry simply because "one o'clock is lunchtime," the arrival of the bread basket at the beginning of a meal), or emotional (comfort eating, the popcorn that makes a movie more of a treat, the tub of ice cream demolished when you're feeling blue). Try, then, to decipher your hunger. Are you really hungry? Or are you overriding your brain's satiety message? Even posing the question can be enough to still the urge.

- **Keep the commitment small**. This is the advice of experimental psychologist Dr. B.J. Fogg at Stanford's brilliantly named Persuasive Technology Lab. According to his research into creating new habits, small steps are more effective than grand gestures: "The number one mistake people make," Fogg told the *Huffington Post*, "is not going tiny enough."[31] If you're trying to make a change in your life, go small. In fact, go minuscule. Make it something that takes almost no effort and nearly no time. "Just put on your running shoes," Fogg says. "That's it. Put them on in the morning every day for five days. You're done." According to Fogg—and it's an appealing proposition— by breaking down each resolution to discover what the smallest constituent habit could be, your chances of succeeding will be 50% higher than if you leave it vague.

- **Know your triggers**. Recognize—before it happens—when your self-control is likely to dissolve. Discover the cue that drives a poor habit, and change the reward. If you're always ravenous when you get home from work, make sure there's an apple stashed in your bag to eat en route, so that you don't demolish a pack of cookies as soon as you're through the front door. Have business lunches in the office or in a park, not in the restaurant where they serve the world's best tiramisu. If you're prone to a late-night forage in the fridge, run a bath instead. Know your food fault-lines—it might be chocolate, ice cream, cheese. In my case, it's dough. For six weeks, commit to a moratorium on your nemesis. Don't buy it. Walk past it. Even demonize it. After six weeks without sugar in your coffee, you may find that the very idea of it makes you shudder. I certainly can't look a latte in the eye these days—even though I was a devoted fan for years before I discovered 5:2.

A Word About Willpower

What do we really know about willpower? It's a slippery beast, the eel of the mind. But recent studies have provided new insights which make stimulating food for thought, and can offer ways to galvanize you during your FastBeach Diet:

- In her book *The Willpower Instinct*, Stanford psychologist Kelly McGonigal suggests that self-control shouldn't be seen as a virtue, but as a muscle: it gets tired from use, but regular exercise makes it stronger. This is great news: it means (as we know from experience on the FastDiet) that the going gets easier if we persevere.

- "Feeling bad" about giving in to a craving only leads to . . . more giving in. It turns out that self-compassion is a far better strategy than self-flagellation. This has long been our approach on the FastDiet, but it's worth being explicit about it here: inner acceptance actually seems to improve outer control—while attempts to fight instincts and desires only serve to make them worse. So, recognizing that thought suppression really doesn't work, make a positive commitment rather than a negative one: instead of saying no, say yes; not "I won't" (eat the muffin), but "I will" (have the apple).

- Similarly, you can "reframe the motivator." Rather than thinking "arrgh, I don't want to be fat," focus on "I'd like to be slimmer, healthier, and full of energy." Consider what you want, frame it positively, write it down and read it every day.

- Self-control is, it seems, subject to social control;[32] we are hardwired to mimic the behavior of others, even when it comes to a pursuit as seemingly solitary as willpower. Psychologists call this "goal contagion," and it resonates with our ideas about embarking on the FastBeach Diet with a friend or a partner, or finding a "goal role model" (you may well discover one at www.thefastdiet.co.uk). You might, for instance, decide to try a reward technique with a friend—each of you could put $10 in a pot; if one of you gives up, both of you lose. Nifty, eh?

    And just add exercise . . .

Chapter 5

Adding Exercise

It won't surprise you to learn that introducing exercise into the FastDiet equation is likely to be hugely beneficial. In conjunction with IF, exercise can help you lose weight (fat, in particular), and it will certainly improve your general fitness, strength, and health—which, never forget, is the overarching goal.

Which Exercise Is Best?

The one you like best. It's the one you'll do.

Even a small amount of "integrative exercise" can really work wonders—studies show that several five-minute bouts of general activity throughout a day will promote cardiovascular and respiratory health, lower your risk of diabetes, and improve your longevity. For some people, it's enough simply to get up and get moving.

If you're up for a greater challenge, now is the time to introduce a more considered exercise plan. Again, commit for the next six weeks, not necessarily beyond. Variety is one of the keys to compliance, so choose two or three different exercises to keep you engaged. It helps if the exercise is time efficient and can fit easily into your day (which is one of the reasons

High Intensity Training gets our vote, as we'll see below). Remember, though, that "exercise" needn't be formal—even a regular, brisk walk will do. You just have to *do it.*

Can I Exercise on a Fast Day?

Yes! Research has shown that even a far more extreme three-day total fast has no negative effect on the ability to perform short-term, high-intensity workouts or longer-duration, moderate-intensity exercise. In fact—and this is worth noting if you already exercise regularly and are aiming for optimal fitness—fasted training can result in "better metabolic adaptations" (which means enhanced performance over time).[33]

If you enjoy cardio workouts, training while fasting can help your body tap into its fat stores—but running a long race on empty is not advised. If you are not used to exercising, then start slowly and listen to your body. During the first week on the FastBeach Diet, novices should limit HIT until they see how their body responds. Some people, incidentally, find that working out the day after a Fast Day can be more challenging; in which case, perhaps make these your rest days to allow your body to adapt to the previous day's efforts.

When Is the Best Time to Exercise?

As readers of *FastExercise* will know, if you are interested in performance, late afternoon or early evening may be a better time to work out. However, sports scientists at Glasgow University found that, while morning exercise may feel harder for some people, it can be a great mood booster, setting you up mentally for the day. Their research showed that women in an 8:15 a.m. aerobics class achieved a 50% boost to their feelings of well-being compared with 20% for those who worked out at 7:15 p.m.[34]

If burning fat is the aim, as we've seen above, you may well find that you benefit from doing exercise in a fasted state. One recent study, for example, found that working out before breakfast is beneficial for metabolic performance and weight loss.[35] According to its authors, "Our current data indicate that exercise training in the fasted state is more effective than exercise in the carbohydrate-fed state."

There is, however, some evidence to suggest gender differences in response to fasted training[36] (men tend to build muscles so long as they work out before their main meal; women tend to respond better to training after a meal). What's more, fasted endurance training may work better for women than fasted weight training.

The truth is we are all different and the best time to exercise is the time that best suits you. What all the experts agree upon is that exercise at any time is better than none at all.

The Two Fundamentals for Fast Fitness

Exercise means different things to different people: a Zumba class, a tennis match, a morning jog around the park. To maximize results on the FastBeach Diet, it's helpful to consider two key areas, and introduce an element of each into your weekly plan:

• Cardio work, particularly HIT

• Strength training for muscle tone

High-Intensity Training (HIT)

Despite increasing evidence to the contrary, there is a persistent belief in the fitness industry that the more time you spend exercising the better. "Go steady but go long" has been the received wisdom, with the promise that you will thus enter the fabled "fat-burning zone." But, as Dr. Stephen Boutcher at the University of New South Wales says, "Most exercise programs designed for weight loss have focused on steady-state exercise of around 30 minutes at a moderate intensity on most days of the week. Disappointingly, these kinds of exercise programs have led to little or no loss".[37]

The latest thinking, developed in several studies and familiar to anyone who has read Michael's *FastExercise* book, is that we can get many of the important benefits of exercise from just three minutes of intense activity a week.[38]

Michael's initial interest in HIT came from meeting Jamie Timmons, a professor of systems biology at Loughborough University. According to Professor Timmons, "The truth about exercise is shocking and intriguing. It's shocking that we've been given such prescriptive guidelines by government, yet have known so little. HIT has blown apart the scientific theories. . . . The work that I and others have done so far suggests that, on average, HIT leads to the same end point as high-volume training. But the key is this: HIT is much easier to do."

Below, you'll find a summary of Michael's approach to HIT. Try it as part of your FastBeach Diet and you'll gain its myriad benefits with only a short, sharp investment of time. If conventional cardio work is more to your taste—whether it's a spin class or a game of squash—by all means commit to doing that. Anything that gets you moving will be a bonus. But I would also encourage you to give HIT a try.

Why Moderate Exercise Gets Mediocre Results

It should be straightforward: do more exercise, burn more calories, lose more weight. The problem is that, when it comes to humans, things are rarely straightforward. Part of the problem is that fat is an incredibly energy-dense substance. A pound of fat contains more energy than a pound of dynamite. This means you have to do a lot of exercise to burn even a small amount of it. Most of us have neither the time nor the inclination to do the quantity of exercise required.

What's more, when we exercise, we tend to engage in "compensatory eating," which rather spoils the plot. Studies show that we often make up for even moderate exercise by eating more.[39] Sometimes a lot more. In fact, the very thought of exercise may encourage us to start eating.[40]

But, if exercise alone is not a great way to lose fat, we do know that combining exercise with a diet is likely to be more effective than either done alone. Over the last decade, studies have repeatedly shown that a few minutes of intense exercise a day can make a huge difference. Unbelievably, there is evidence that just 40 seconds of intense activity can have a significant effect.[41]

As Michael discovered, you really can get many of the same benefits, perhaps more, from doing HIT as you can from slogging away at the more traditional approach.

These benefits include:

• Improved aerobic fitness and endurance

• Reduced body fat

• Increased body strength

The studies show that:

• HIT will get you aerobically fitter faster than standard exercise

• HIT will improve insulin sensitivity faster than standard exercise

• If you want to build muscle tone and lose some fat, HIT will be the most time-efficient way to go about it

How Does HIT Burn Fat?

When you push the intensity of a workout, you build more metabolically active muscle, and, because muscle is efficient at burning fat, your total calorie expenditure soars. This happens mainly because HIT encourages the muscle cells to produce new mitochondria, the power plants that transfer fat into energy and heat. The mitochondria not only burn fat when you are exercising, but go on doing so for some time afterwards as your muscles recover.

The metabolic stress caused by HIT also leads to an increase in the production of "catecholamines"—hormones such as adrenaline and noradrenaline—which lead to much greater fat burning. There are more catecholamine receptors in abdominal fat than in subcutaneous fat, so when you get a surge of catecholamines following a vigorous burst of HIT, they target abdominal fat, increasing the release of fat from visceral fat stores.

HIT and Insulin Sensitivity

Professor Timmons tested Michael for a number of health indices before he started his HIT program, and then, after four weeks, he returned to the lab to be retested. One of the main tests was for insulin sensitivity (Michael, as readers of *The FastDiet* will know, was particularly interested in this result as his father died from complications linked to diabetes).

At his first testing, Michael's insulin sensitivity result showed he was just within what is regarded as healthy tolerance. Timmons pointed to several studies which showed that doing just three minutes of HIT a week could improve insulin sensitivity by 24%. And this is exactly the amount by which Michael's own index improved. Other studies have shown even greater improvements in insulin sensitivity following an HIT regimen. One found a 35% improvement in insulin sensitivity after only two weeks.[42]

So why is this relevant on your FastBeach Diet? Insulin sensitivity is what keeps your blood glucose stable. As we've seen in chapter 4, when you eat, your digestive system releases glucose into your bloodstream; this causes the pancreas to release insulin, a hormone that triggers body tissue to absorb circulating glucose. Reduced insulin sensitivity means that the pancreas has to release more and more insulin to keep blood-sugar levels stable. Abnormally low insulin sensitivity is known as "insulin resistance," a condition that results in high levels of insulin, glucose, and fats circulating in the bloodstream. This is a main risk factor for metabolic syndrome, which increases the risk of coronary artery disease, stroke, and type 2 diabetes.

It is not yet clear precisely how HIT affects insulin sensitivity, but Timmons and some other scientists suggest it could be because HIT uses many more muscles than conventional aerobic training. HIT engages 80% of the muscles of the body, compared to around 30–40% during moderate jogging or cycling. One of the effects of exercise is to break down glycogen, a stored form of glucose, in muscles. Removing stores of glycogen makes way for fresh glucose to be taken up from the bloodstream. So the more muscle tissue engaged in exercise, the more space is available for new glucose deposits. As Michael wrote in *FastExercise*, vigorous exercise such as HIT creates "a much bigger sink for the glucose that follows a meal."

HIT and Appetite Suppression

HIT also seems to suppress appetite in ways that low intensity exercise does not. One study showed that young men ate fewer calories after high-intensity workouts than they did after a bout of moderate exercise.[43] Even more encouragingly, the men reported eating fewer calories on the day *following* the highest intensity workout than they did after the moderate session or after resting. So one of their most striking findings is that if you do very high-intensity exercise, the effects of appetite suppression last far longer, well into the next day.

HIT, Your Way

The joy of FastExercise (and what it has in common with the FastDiet) is that the exertion is only short-lived: it's the perfect workout for the time-starved generation. As we've established, any exercise at all is better than none. But if you want to introduce HIT into your six-week plan, here's how to go about it:

• The exact choice of exercise is yours. You may already have a favorite activity or gym session. Now's the time to turn up the dial.

• The aim is to do three sessions a week; the temptation may be to do more. Don't.

• Remember, this is about quality, not quantity. Effort is more important than the amount of time you spend or the number of repetitions you do. Try any of the following:

Outdoor Running

To turn a normal run into an HIT session, you'll have to inject real intensity into your workout, which means including a few sprints, preferably up a hill. Uphill sprinting is one of the most effective forms of HIT, but if you are not especially fit, build up to this gradually.

• Warm up by jogging for 1–2 minutes
• Run flat-out up a hill for 10 seconds
• Recover for 1–2 minutes
• Repeat

Increase to three or four 30-second bouts as you get fitter. After running up a hill, avoid jogging back down; walk down instead.

Indoor Running

Running on a treadmill burns about 5% fewer calories than running outdoors, due to the lack of wind resistance and because the motorized belt helps to propel you along. So crank up the gradient to make sure you are working hard enough.

Follow the protocol for running outdoors, with warm-up, 10-second bouts, and recovery—building up the incline and sprint time as you get fitter.

Indoor Cycling

• Pedal gently for 1–2 minutes with the resistance on a low setting
• Then set the resistance level to your limit and go to your maximum effort level for 20 seconds

• Pedal gently again for another 1–2 minutes to allow your heart rate to return to normal.
• Repeat

If you are unfit or have never tried HIT before, start with two 10-second sprints and build up to two 20-second sprints over several weeks. Increase resistance by 2% every two weeks. Advance to three or four 20-second bouts as you get fitter.

Stair Running

This is fairly low impact on the knees and feet, and great for buttock and leg toning. You'll need several flights of stairs, so perhaps try this at work.

• Bound up stairs for 30 seconds
• Recover for 1–2 minutes
• Repeat

The whole foot should land on the stair, and don't run downstairs. You can, of course, do this on a step machine.

Cross-training

• Warm up for 1–2 minutes
• Set to the highest incline and resistance and go at maximum effort for 20 seconds
• Recover for 1-2 minutes
• Repeat and build up to three reps and 30-second bouts as your fitness improves

Swimming

Swimming is a superlative all-around workout and will give you a defined waist and strong shoulders, but it's important to vary the strokes. Rather than judge by time, judge by distance. A 25-metre length at full intensity is comparable to sprinting for around 30–40 seconds.

- Warm up at a leisurely pace for a length
- "Sprint swim" for half a length
- Recover for 1–2 minutes
- Repeat

Again, build up the sprinting distance and reps to three rounds as you get fitter.

FOOD AND FAST EXERCISE

- Don't attempt FastExercise immediately after eating: the main risk is not cramping but vomiting
- Don't load up on carbs before doing FastExercise. There is a widespread belief that carbs are needed to fuel exercise. Unless you are exercising heavily for over an hour at a time, you have plenty of carbohydrates on board.
- Similarly, you don't need to load up on carbs after doing FastExercise either. You may feel a bit wobbly but, as we've seen above, the point of doing HIT is to deplete your glycogen reserves (the energy stored

in your muscles), making way for fresh glucose to be deposited in the bloodstream, so the last thing you want to do is immediately replenish them. The average person doing a HIT session three times a week does not require special "refueling."

IS HIT SAFE?

Michael suggests that if you are unfit you should ease yourself into HIT. Don't exercise if you feel unwell; your body needs its resources to get better. Anyone who has doubts about their health should have a medical checkup before starting any form of exercise.

Strength Training

Of course, getting fit is about more than simply doing cardiovascular exercise, whether you take a traditional approach or try HIT. A beach-fit body requires tone and flexibility too. Weight training while fasting can help your body build more lean muscle (particularly if you are male) and maintain bone density. It will give you a lengthened, strengthened figure—exactly what you want as you head for the beach with only a swimsuit for company. The following simple, familiar exercises are just suggestions; you may well have your own favorites. Since you don't need any special equipment—just the resistance of your own body weight— you can do them anywhere, any time. You could do them now. Include some or all of the following exercises, adapted from fitness expert Peta Bee's program in *FastExercise*, on the days when you're not doing HIT.

Push-ups

Lie face down with the palms of your hands directly beneath your shoulders and the balls of your feet touching the ground. Keep your body straight—your head in line with your back—and raise yourself up using your arms. Lower your torso to the ground until your elbows form a 90-degree angle and then push up again. If you find this too challenging, do it with your knees on the ground until you are strong enough to perform full push-ups.

Jumping Jacks or Star Jumps

You'll remember these from PE lessons at school, and there's something joyful about doing them in the kitchen while you're waiting for the kettle to boil. Stand with your hands by your sides. In one movement, jump up with your legs apart as you raise your arms to the sides. Land with your arms over your head and your feet more than hip-width apart. Jump up again and, in one movement, bring your legs together and your hands back to your sides.

Wall Sit

Start with your back against a wall with your feet shoulder-width apart and positioned about two feet from the wall. Slowly slide your back down the wall until your thighs are parallel to the ground and your knees are directly above your ankles. Don't arch your back. Hold the position for as long as you can.

Ab Crunches

Lie on your back with your knees bent, your feet flat on the floor, and your hands positioned on either side of your head. Raise your upper body without lifting your lower back off the ground, making sure your chin is tucked in toward your chest. When your shoulders and upper back are lifted off the floor, gently curl back down.

Squats

Stand with your feet shoulder-width apart and hands placed lightly on opposite shoulders. Imagine you are preparing to sit in a chair; bend at the knee, keeping the weight on your heels. Make sure your back is as straight as possible. Keep bending until your legs make a 90-degree angle, with your thighs parallel to the ground. Push back up without bending your back.

Plank

Lie on your front on the floor and then raise yourself onto your forearms and toes so that your body forms a straight line from head to toe. Make sure your midsection doesn't lift or drop. Hold the position for as long as possible. Remember, it should never cause pain in your lower back.

Lunges

Stand with your back straight and your feet shoulder-width apart. Stride forward with one leg, bending both knees to 90 degrees and keeping your upper body straight. Pull back to the starting position and repeat with the other leg.

Do as many repeats of each exercise as you can manage in 30 seconds and take a 10-second rest between each bout. Again, over the six weeks, aim to increase the number of reps, and/or the length of each bout.

FINDING FLEXIBILITY AND STRENGTH
THROUGH YOGA AND PILATES

Yoga and Pilates, among their many benefits, will bless you with a stronger, leaner body. They also aid posture, balance, and core strength. Dynamic yoga such as Ashtanga or Bikram will give you a more intense workout, but regular practice of any form will help strengthen and define muscles, particularly if you hold the poses—downward dog, plank, and chaturanga dandasana (a yogic push-up) can be challenging and intense, particularly as a dynamic sequence in the sun salutation. Yoga will also put you in touch with your body, something that can get overlooked when we reside mainly in the mind. Noticing (not judging) how your body feels and reacts on any given day, right now, is the basis of good yoga practice and a crucial starting point for the FastDiet. Including meditation and breathing practice will support your mindfulness mission. As a yoga nut with 20 years of practice behind me, I strongly advise that you find a teacher who speaks your language and inspires you. Pilates, too, will help streamline a body. You'll gain spine mobility and core strength, together with improved skeletal alignment. All good.

Everyday Exercise: What to Do When on the FastBeach Diet

Aim to introduce HIT three times a week. You can choose which days—as we've seen, there's no reason to avoid exercise on a Fast Day. But find a balance that seems to work for you. Again, apply the motivator that this is just for six weeks: it's a means to an end. You may well find that exercise, in whatever form, soon becomes an integral and enjoyable part of your life.

On two other days, introduce strengthening exercises whenever and wherever you can. Five minutes of push-ups and planks before bed. A half-hour yoga session before you start work. Lunges and crunches in front of your favorite TV show. Whatever you can do, do. Just ensure that you have two rest days, free of exercise.

How to Bring Exercise into Your Life

It's all very well to make a plan. But how to make it happen? Sometimes, as we discovered when looking at habits in chapter 4, it's enough to shift your perspective by doing small, seemingly inconsequential things:

- **Put on your workout clothes, not jeans, first thing—** and keep your sneakers handy. Just as you are more likely to eat chips if they're in full view, so you are more likely to exercise if the cues are staring you in the face. Put your running shoes by the front door, move the exercise bike into the family room; find somewhere else to hang your washing other than on the cross-trainer. As Dr. Fogg's investigations have shown, tiny steps such as these can change the clockwork routine of your day.

- **Write a pledge, and make it as specific as you can.** "I will do a 5-minute session of HIT on the exercise bike, three times a week starting tomorrow evening when I get back from work" would be a good start. Pin it on the wall, schedule it into your diary, put reminders on your phone, tell your kids. Whatever works for you, but the more clearly you have thought it through, the more likely you are to do it.

- **Write a list of potential excuses.** Can't find shoes, running clothes in the wash, I'm tired, it's cold, football's on the telly . . . Now address each in turn and write down the solutions. Anticipating potential barriers reduces the chance of backsliding.

- **Monitor your progress.** Remember the power of positive feedback? Remember the benefits of keeping a food diary and logging your achievements? The same goes for exercise.

Download an app that appeals to you (the FastBeach Diet app will help you track your workouts), or use the pull-out planner included in this book.

- **Take advantage of your environment**. Use that park bench, tackle that hill. Or you could simply embrace one of Michael's pet projects and *always take the stairs*. Some time ago, I came across a comment from British architect Will Alsop: "If you really wanted to do something about [the obesity crisis]," he said, "You could take all the elevators out of all the buildings in London. Then people would be fit."[44] He's not wrong. When employees of the University Hospital of Geneva were banned from using the lift for 12 weeks—a move that increased their daily climb from five to 23 flights of stairs—their aerobic capacity increased by an average of 8.6% and their body-fat levels fell by 2%.[45]

- **Get up, get out, get going**. We apparently spend an average of 14 hours and 28 minutes a day sitting down— the equivalent of 36 years of our adult lives.[46] Allowing for eight hours' sleep, we spend a meager hour and a half on our feet, active, each day. Researchers have found that, after a day without movement, lipase, an enzyme that helps the body break down fat, is suppressed, almost to the point of shutting off. When we sit, fat is more likely to be stored as adipose tissue than be passed to the muscles where it can be burned. Sitting for prolonged periods thus results in the retention of fat, a lower HDL (that's the "good cholesterol"), and an overall reduction in the metabolic rate.[47]

So, try a few tiny tricks to make a stand:

• Go and see a colleague instead of sending an email.

• Stand up and pace about while talking on the phone.

• Drink plenty of water. This not only keeps you hydrated but it also increases the need for bathroom breaks, which means in turn more short, brisk walks.

• Have a car-free week: a study of 11,000 Atlanta residents reported a correlation between driving and weight gain, with every additional hour spent in a car each day associated with a 6% increase in the likelihood of obesity.[48] For the next six weeks, leave the car at home whenever you can.

• Tell people. Publicly stating a goal makes you more likely to follow through, especially, it seems, if you are female.

• Exercise with others. If you're planning on going for a jog or a walk, invite someone to do it with you. One of the main reasons people employ personal trainers is to have someone to get them out of the house when they don't feel like going.

• Get a gadget. Pedometer use is associated with significant increases in physical activity and decreases in BMI and blood pressure.[49] Fitness apps—you could try the Fast Exercise app—are likely to have a similar effect.

Exercise and its benefits are all in the body, right? But what if they're also in the mind? A fabulous piece of research in this area came from Harvard's psychology department in 2007.[50] It involved 84 female hotel attendants from seven hotels, each of whom cleaned an average of 15 rooms a day. Despite this being hard, physical labor, 66% of the women reported that they did not exercise regularly. More than 36% said they got no exercise at all.

The researchers then divided them into two groups, giving one group detailed information about the calorie burn and health benefits of the activities such as vacuuming and cleaning that they undertook every day. After a month, the tutored group perceived that they did more exercise than before, while the untutored group's responses were unchanged. Neither group had altered their actual level of activity.

But here's the fascinating bit: despite no change in exercise level, the tutored group showed "improvement on every single one of the objective health measures recorded: weight, body fat, body mass index, waist-to-hip ratio and blood pressure." They had lost an average of 2 pounds and lowered their blood pressure by almost 10%. Just something to think about the next time you pull on your running shoes for a session of HIT . . .

Chapter 6

My FastBeach Diet Diary

So, now that you have a real feel for the FastBeach Diet, it's time to get down to the nitty-gritty. What happens on a day-to-day basis? What can you expect? Here's a typical "week in the life" of the FastBeach Diet for me, together with approximate calorie counts (your schedule will, of course, differ, but notice the efforts I've made to take in as much exercise and as many "good" habits as possible).

Sunday
Non-Fast Day
HIT Day 1

Morning: toast and honey (I have whole grain bread and stop at one slice rather than my habitual two), peppermint tea, half a mango with lime

Afternoon: Sunday lunch with the family at the pub (I order a child's portion of roast beef and don't have dessert), followed by a proper, long walk with the dog on the Downs; we race each other to the top of the hill.

Evening: I'm not particularly hungry in the evening, so I have veggie soup from the freezer, with a slice of whole grain bread and a bit of goat cheese. Once the kids are in bed, instead of watching TV, I do a HIT session on the exercise bike. *Then* I watch TV.

Total calories: approximately 1,600—no need to count every calorie, just be gently "aware"
Total exercise: long walk and HIT

Monday
Fast Day 1

Morning: oatmeal and berries for breakfast, black coffee; half an hour of stretching and strength exercises

Afternoon: No lunch. I'm a bit hungry, so I eat an apple, seeds and all. More black coffee, peppermint tea. Busy at work, time flies.

Evening: Harissa-spiced chicken breast with a huge pile of salad—lots of different leaves and seeds. Early to bed; tomorrow's another day.

Total calories: 500
Total exercise: stretching and strength exercises

Tuesday
Non-Fast Day

Morning: Scrambled eggs and a whole grain tortilla for breakfast. I take the dog for a brisk walk along the beach, walking fast enough to be slightly out of breath.

Afternoon: Out for lunch with friends. I walk rather than drive, just for a change (no parking fee!). I order baked cod with cherry tomatoes and French green lentils, no bread, no dessert. Sparkling water with fresh lime.

Evening: Pilates class 6 p.m. Family dinner of spaghetti Bolognese. I have a small portion, and fill half of my plate with vegetables—broccoli, sugar snap peas. Plain yogurt with toasted hazelnuts and a swirl of honey.

Total calories: around 1,700—again, no need to be particular about counting
Total exercise: walking the dog, walking all day (no car), Pilates class

Wednesday
Non-Fast Day
HIT Day 2
Meat-free day

Morning: oatmeal with cinnamon and nuts for breakfast, black coffee, water

Afternoon: A busy day at work, so I have lunch at my desk: sashimi and edamame from Yo! Sushi and a packet of miso soup, plus plenty of sparkling water.

Evening: Not as hungry as I was expecting. I have cauliflower gratin for dinner, but no crispy bacon. I don't have seconds. Half a cantaloupe, some blueberries, and handful of almonds. A session of HIT—uphill running, 15 minutes—followed by half an hour of yoga.

Total calories: around 1,200
Total exercise: HIT session, half-an-hour of yoga

Thursday
Fast Day 2

Morning: I have an early work meeting so I arrange to have it on the move down by the seafront, not at a restaurant. No breakfast, but plenty of water and chamomile tea.

Afternoon: No lunch.

Evening: Tuscan summer bean soup and a small portion of Thai beef salad (see chapter 7). Stretching and strength exercises (jumping jacks, push-ups, and planks), half an hour of yoga, then early to bed.

Total calories: 525
Total exercise: walk along the seafront, take stairs not elevators all day, stretching and strengthening exercises, yoga

Friday
Non-Fast Day

Morning: Breakfast on the go as I have to catch an early train—small fruit salad and instant oatmeal, black coffee from Pret.

Afternoon: No time for proper lunch, but grab some flatbread, an apple, and Gruyère cheese; plenty of sparkling water. Don't take the subway, but walk between meetings. Take the stairs (quickly) at the station. I buy a green juice on the way home.

Evening: Takeout curry with the family. I have a chicken tikka with plain rice, not pilaf, and tarka dahl (lentils) and okra. No naan.

Total calories: around 1,700
Total exercise: stair climbing and pavement walking

Saturday
Non-Fast Day
HIT Day 3

Morning: Quick session of HIT before breakfast to see what "fasted training" feels like. Quite hungry afterwards, but make a point of not eating fast-release carbs. Have poached eggs on slice of toast, followed by yogurt and chopped pear. Black coffee.

Afternoon: Dog walk on the Downs. Lunch with the kids—we have a tricolore salad—avocado, mozzarella, cherry tomatoes, and baby spinach leaves. I leave the bread and dessert to the children, but have a small handful of grapes and pistachios with my peppermint tea.

Evening: Out with friends—decide not to stay out for dinner (I have grilled salmon with green beans and olives—"O'Kelly fish"—at home) and go to the movies instead. I drink water, not soda, and share a small bar of Green & Black's Maya Gold chocolate (rather than buying the big size).

Total calories: around 1,600
Total exercise: HIT bike session, dog walking

You'll notice that there's no alcohol and not many snacks on my list. Remember, this plan is only six weeks long. You can do it.

Chapter 7

The Recipes

Simple Summer Food . . . The Perfect Fit for the FastBeach Diet

Like many people, I find fasting so much easier in summer. Not only are the fresh seasonal ingredients perfect for Fast Day dishes, the heat (when it comes) also serves to take the edge off your appetite. Most of us don't hunger for carbs and cake when the temperature rises; what we're after are sharp, clean flavors and snappy cooking, the kind that lets us spend more time outdoors and less time glued to the stove.

In summer, plenty of FastDieters will eat simple grilled fish or meat—perhaps marinated in chili peppers and spice, or lemon and herbs—alongside a great mass of salad leaves or steamed greens. Others prefer to embark on something with a bit more pizazz. The recipes here will broaden your repertoire and give your mouth something to think about on a Fast Day. But first, what's for breakfast?

Breakfast

Fast Day Muesli
120 calories per 1-ounce portion

Try making your own low-GI muesli with plenty of seeds and nuts. It's satiating and tasty, but quite caloric (blame the nuts), so use sparingly, more as a topping than a base. And stick with it: once you've trained your taste buds to enjoy this infinitely superior Fast Day version, the store-bought sugared varieties won't compare.

- 3.5 ounces rolled oats
- 3.5 ounces rye flakes
- 1 ounce oat bran
- 2 tablespoons each sunflower seeds, pumpkin seeds, flax seeds, poppy seeds
- 2 tablespoons each almonds and hazelnuts, coarsely chopped
- 2 tablespoons coconut flakes (for sweetness)

Combine the ingredients—this makes about 12.5 ounces—and keep the muesli in an airtight container (you can, of course, multiply the quantities).

Fast Day Muesli with Fresh Strawberries and Yogurt
245 calories per portion
Serves 1

    1 ounce Fast Day muesli
    3.5 ounces low-fat plain yogurt
    10 strawberries

Add a handful of muesli to yogurt and top with strawberries.

Oat Berry Smoothie
220 calories per portion
Serves 1

Oats are full of soluble fiber and release energy slowly to set you up for the day (use rolled oats rather than the more finely milled varieties).

    5 ounces skim milk
    3.5 ounces low-fat Greek yogurt
    3 tablespoons rolled oats
    1.7 ounces raspberries or blueberries

Put all ingredients in a blender and blitz. Alternatively, leave out the berries (-25 calories) and try the oat base with:

- Chopped dates (+46 calories for two) and apricots (+24 calories for three halves of dried fruit)
- Honey (+22 calories per teaspoon) and 1 tablespoon fresh blackberries (+15 calories)
- Chopped pear (+103 calories per medium pear) and nutmeg
- Apple (+72 calories per medium apple), cinnamon, and vanilla extract
- Banana (+105 calories) and honey (+22 calories per teaspoon)

Another way to add sweetness is to use lactose-free cow's milk, which is slightly sweeter on the palate than regular milk. Or try almond milk for a nondairy alternative.

Scrambled Eggs
220 calories per portion
Serves 1

  2 medium eggs
  1 tablespoon milk (optional)
  ½ teaspoon butter
  Sea salt and pepper

Beat the eggs with milk, sea salt, and freshly ground pepper. Whisk well. Melt butter in a small nonstick pan and cook very gently, constantly stirring. Remove from heat.

Serve with . . .

- Smoked salmon (+90 calories for 1.7 ounces) or flakes of hot smoked trout (+70 calories for 1.7 ounces)
- Turmeric, cumin, finely chopped green onion, a little green chili pepper, and a chopped ripe tomato (+20 calories)
- Mustard (+15 calories per tablespoon)
- Pesto (+135 calories per tablespoon), a crumble of feta (+69 calories for .8 ounce) and a sprinkle of fresh basil leaves
- Torn watercress and a dash of balsamic vinegar
- A handful of arugula and sliced bell peppers (+12 calories for 1.7 ounces)
- Parmesan (+60 calories for .6 ounce) and anchovies (+20 calories for 4 drained fillets)—grate the cheese, chop the fish, add to the egg mixture before cooking
- Shrimp (+36 calories for 1.7 ounces) and cilantro

Poached Eggs

180 calories per portion
Serves 1

  2 medium eggs
  1 teaspoon white wine vinegar

Boil a large pot of lightly salted water and keep at a simmer over gentle heat. Crack a medium egg into a cup. Swirl the simmering water, add vinegar to help the egg white coagulate;

then gently add the egg. Poach for 2 to 3 minutes, or until set to your liking. Remove from the pot with a slotted spoon and set it to dry on paper towels.

Serve with . . .

- Prosciutto: trimmed of fat (+80 calories for 2 slices)
- Spinach: loosely chopped. Heat 2 tablespoons of butter (+75 calories) in a small frying pan and sauté for a minute. Perhaps add a pinch of red pepper flakes, a finely sliced green onion, and a squeeze of lemon (which will help the vitamins in the spinach to be absorbed).
- Smoked herring fillets: to cook with no smell, place fish in a microwaveable dish, add a slice of lemon, cover with plastic wrap, and microwave for 2½ minutes, or until cooked through (+232 calories for 3.5 ounces).

Boiled Eggs
90 calories per egg
Serves 1

Take a medium egg, place in a pot of cold water, bring to a boil, and allow to simmer for 3 to 4 minutes, or until cooked to your liking.

Serve with . . .

- Asparagus spears: trim 5 asparagus spears and either add to the boiling water with the egg, or steam for 3 to 4 minutes

---

Tricolore Omelet
184 calories per portion (216 with cheese)
Serves 1

Go for goat cheese if you can, as it has fewer calories and less fat than the average cheese made from cow's milk: 80 calories and 6 grams of fat per ounce, compared to around 100 calories and 10 grams of fat per ounce. This is a fine way to get punch and flavor into what could be a bland dish; include the cheese to get the full taste and tricolore effect, but leave it out if calories are scarce.

    1 green onion, finely chopped
    ½ teaspoon red pepper flakes
    Cooking spray
    2 medium eggs
    Salt and pepper
    .3 ounce goat cheese (optional)
    Curly parsley, chopped

Lightly fry the green onion and red pepper flakes (as many or as few as you fancy) in a small frying pan with just a spray of oil to prevent sticking. Beat the eggs with a fork until bubbly. Add salt and plenty of pepper, and cook gently until the omelet is set to your liking. Add a crumble of goat cheese, if using, and the parsley to serve.

Dinner

Fish

Deb's Monkfish with Roasted Peppers and Tomatoes
289 calories per portion
Serves 2

Monkfish tends to be fairly expensive, but this is one of those dishes with a bit of drama and delight. A Fast Day Special . . .

   2 monkfish fillets (about 7 ounces each)
   4 ripe tomatoes
   2 teaspoons olive oil
   2 tablespoons balsamic vinegar
   Sea salt and black pepper
   1 garlic clove, finely chopped
   2 red peppers, left whole
   Handful of fresh basil leaves
   4 slices of prosciutto, fat removed

Preheat the oven to 350°F. Slice the tomatoes crosswise and place on a baking sheet. Drizzle with the olive oil and balsamic vinegar, season, and dot with the garlic. Place the peppers in the baking sheet alongside the tomatoes. Roast for 30 minutes, until softened and slightly charred. Set tomatoes aside, and place peppers in a bowl. Cover with plastic wrap and allow to steam. Once cooled, remove the skin and seeds, then cut into wide strips.

Clean the monkfish fillets, removing any membrane, and dry well. Gently season them. Place 4 or 5 strips of roasted pepper on one fillet, and top with 4 or 5 basil leaves. Lay the remaining fillet on top and wrap the parcel firmly in prosciutto, securing with toothpicks if necessary.

Cook in the hot oven for 20 to 25 minutes, or until cooked through (this will depend on size and thickness of the fish; check after 20 minutes). Let rest for 5 to 10 minutes. Meanwhile, put the remaining peppers, roasted tomatoes, and more fresh basil in a blender and puree. Either serve at room temperature, or warm the puree in a small saucepan on a low heat; season to taste. Slice the fish into four medallions and serve drizzled with pepper puree. A salad of soft leaves would be nice too.

Italian Seafood Salad

261 calories per portion
Serves 4

Lightly poached seafood makes an ideal, and incredibly simple, Fast Day dinner. Buy it fresh or frozen, cook it quickly, and serve at once.

As an alternative, this salad is just as good with an Asian kick—just use chopped cilantro instead of parsley and chives, lime juice to replace the lemon, and a mix of sesame oil and olive oil. A sprinkle of sesame seeds would seal the deal.

14 ounces raw shell-on shrimp
14 ounces mussels
14 ounces squid rings

For the dressing
Juice of a lemon
2 tablespoons extra-virgin olive oil
1 garlic clove, crushed
1 tablespoon flat-leaf parsley, coarsely chopped
1 tablespoon chives, snipped
¼ teaspoon red pepper flakes (or more to taste)
Sea salt and freshly ground pepper

For the salad
1 red onion, very thinly sliced
1 bag of baby lettuce leaves

Mix the dressing ingredients and set aside. Bring a large saucepan of water to a boil, add seafood—the squid last as it cooks the quickest—and simmer for 2 minutes, or until just cooked through. Drain and discard any mussels that have not opened during cooking. Remove the mussels from their shells and peel the shrimp. Place all the seafood in a bowl and pour dressing over it. Chill for 30 minutes and add to the salad ingredients. Serve with lemon slices.

Clara's Shrimp on Toast
310 calories per portion
Serves 2

I don't usually add unnecessary carbs to a Fast Day recipe, but here, the ciabatta is a worthwhile addition—mainly because it acts as a sponge, soaking up all those tangy flavors. You can, of course, leave it out if you prefer.

10.5 ounces shelled jumbo shrimp, cooked

For the dressing
1 teaspoon grated fresh ginger
2 garlic cloves, finely chopped
1 green chili pepper, seeded and finely chopped
   (more or less to taste)
Handful of fresh cilantro, chopped
Handful of basil leaves, chopped
Juice of half a lemon
2 tablespoons extra-virgin olive oil
Sea salt and freshly ground pepper

2 slices of ciabatta to serve

Combine shrimp and dressing ingredients and refrigerate for 30 minutes. Toast ciabatta and top with the shrimp mixture. Serve.

If you have calories to spare, half a chopped avocado would be welcome in the mix. Add 120 calories per portion.

Sticky Fish with Ginger, Lime, and Zucchini Salad

335 calories per portion with salmon; 219 calories with white fish
Serves 2

This works well with most fish—but is probably best friends with salmon, which happens to have a higher calorie count than white fish. In terms of sustainability, you can't beat tilapia, but take advice from your fishmonger about what is the best fish to place on this bed of herby, tangy vegetables.

2 fish fillets (about 3.5 ounces each)

For the sauce
1 red chili pepper, very finely chopped
1 teaspoon grated fresh ginger
2 teaspoons honey
½ garlic clove, crushed
½ lemongrass stalk, tender heart only, very finely
   chopped
2 green onions, finely sliced
2 teaspoons Thai fish sauce
2 teaspoons soy sauce
Salt and pepper

For the salad
2 small zucchini, peeled into long ribbons
3.5 ounces bean sprouts

Handful cilantro
Handful mint leaves

Preheat oven to 350°F. Mix sauce ingredients. Season fish fillets, place in a small roasting pan and spoon 2 teaspoons of the sauce on top of each. Bake for 15 minutes, or until cooked to your liking. Combine salad ingredients with the remaining sauce. Serve alongside the baked fish, drizzled with any further juices from the pan.

Salmon Tartare, Raw and Smoked
282 calories per portion
Serves 1

The combination of raw and smoked here is truly delicious, and rather sophisticated too. Dill, with its delicate green tendrils and mild anise flavor, is an ideal companion; it must be fresh, though. Dried dill is a dead loss.

3.5 ounces raw salmon fillet, very fresh, chilled, and
   finely chopped
2 teaspoons soy sauce
½ teaspoon grated fresh ginger
1.7 ounces smoked salmon, finely chopped

For the dressing
2 teaspoons lemon juice

Lemon zest
2 tablespoons low-fat plain yogurt
Snipped chives and chopped dill leaves
1 teaspoon capers, rinsed and finely chopped
Dill to garnish

Mix the raw salmon with soy sauce and ginger, cover, and set aside in fridge to marinate for 10 minutes. Add smoked salmon and return the mixture to the fridge. Mix dressing ingredients. Spoon the dressing over the chilled tartare, and top with a generous scattering of dill.

Meat

Spiced Chicken with Warm Lentils and Roasted Garlic
399 calories per portion
Serves 4

A hearty, tasty dish that's good to eat with friends on a warm summer evening. Don't be alarmed by the quantity of garlic—it softens and sweetens during cooking and adds an unctuous, squashy quality to proceedings.

For the marinade
1 teaspoon grated fresh ginger

1 teaspoon ground coriander

1 teaspoon ground cumin

1 teaspoon paprika

1 teaspoon ground turmeric

Juice of a lemon

2 teaspoons olive oil

Salt and pepper

1 medium chicken (about 3 pounds)

1 head of garlic, sliced crosswise

4 ounces French green lentils, rinsed

2 tablespoons water

Generous handful of parsley, chopped

Generous handful of cilantro leaves, chopped

1 tablespoon snipped chives

Juice of half a lemon

Sea salt and freshly ground pepper

Whisk marinade ingredients together and rub into chicken, working under the skin. Refrigerate for 1 hour, or overnight if possible. Preheat oven to 350°F. Place chicken and garlic in a roasting pan and roast for 1 hour 10 minutes—or until the juices run clear. Remove garlic and chicken from oven and allow to rest on a separate plate, retaining the juices in the pan. While the chicken is cooking, place lentils in a saucepan, cover with water and boil; when cooked but still al dente, drain and rinse with cold water, drain again and add them to the roasting pan along with 2 tablespoons water. Heat through, scraping the pan for tasty, sticky bits on the base. Remove from heat and add herbs and lemon juice. Stir well, season, and serve in a generous mound with the carved or torn chicken (with skin removed) and soft garlic.

Chicken and Mango Salad
418 calories per portion
Serves 2

A light, bright, and totally tasty update on chicken salad—made in minutes and probably demolished in seconds (though I would advise relishing every forkful).

  8 small chicken fillets (about 10 ounces total)
  Olive oil cooking spray
  1 teaspoon curry powder (mild, medium, or hot, to taste)

  For the dressing
  4 tablespoons low-fat Greek yogurt (2% fat)
  2 tablespoons mango chutney
  1 teaspoon curry powder
  Zest and juice of a lime
  2 teaspoons water (if you prefer a runnier dressing)
  Salt and pepper

  For the salad
  2 romaine hearts

3.5 ounces sugar snap peas, blanched for 2 minutes in
    boiling water and rinsed with cold water
1 ripe mango, peeled and sliced
½ small red onion, very finely sliced
1 green chili pepper, seeded and finely chopped
Handful of cilantro, coarsely chopped

Heat oven to 350°F. Spray the chicken pieces with a little olive oil, season and dust with curry powder. Place in a small foil-lined baking sheet and bake for 10 to 15 minutes, until cooked through. Once slightly cooled, tear or slice into bite-size pieces. Combine dressing ingredients in a bowl and add the cooked chicken. Assemble the salad ingredients, top with the chicken mixture, and sprinkle with fresh cilantro.

Lime and Herb Chicken Salad
195 calories per portion
Serves 1

Just about my favorite Fast Day food. This is what it's all about: minimum calories, maximum taste.

1 small chicken breast, skin on
A little olive oil
Salt and pepper
½ small cucumber, cut in half lengthwise, seeded,
    cut on the diagonal into crescents

Handful cilantro, including finely chopped stalks
Handful mint leaves
1½ tablespoons Thai fish sauce
1 tablespoon lime juice
1 green onion, finely sliced on the diagonal
½ teaspoon Szechuan peppercorns, crushed
½ teaspoon sesame oil
Iceberg lettuce (2.8 ounces), torn
Lime wedges

Preheat the oven to 350°F. Season chicken and rub it lightly with the oil. Bake until cooked through and juices run clear—about 20 minutes. Let rest. Remove the skin, tear chicken into shreds, and place in a bowl with cucumber, cilantro, and mint. Stir in fish sauce, lime juice, green onion, Szechuan peppercorns, and sesame oil. Toss well. Serve on torn iceberg lettuce and garnish with lime wedges and cilantro leaves.

Thai Beef Salad
351 calories per portion
Serves 2

One we know and love, but an ideal choice for a quick, filling, and (most crucially) pleasing Fast Day summer dinner. Keep the beef rare and thinly sliced. If you're eating with friends, multiply the quantities and perhaps cook your steak on the barbecue.

12 ounces sirloin steak, cut thick and trimmed of fat
(ask your butcher)
Juice of half a lime
1 teaspoon brown sugar
Sea salt
Szechuan peppercorns, ground

For the dressing
2 tablespoons lime juice
2 tablespoons Thai fish sauce
1 teaspoon soy sauce
1 garlic clove, crushed
1 lemongrass stalk, outer leaves removed, finely
chopped
1 bird's eye chili pepper, seeded and finely sliced
(to taste)
2 green onions, finely sliced on the diagonal
Handful of cilantro leaves, coarsely chopped
1 teaspoon brown sugar

For the salad
1 head romaine lettuce, leaves washed and torn
2 ripe tomatoes, cut into eighths (skins removed if
you prefer)
½ cucumber, cut in half lengthwise, seeded, and
sliced into crescents
1 medium red onion, thinly sliced
Handful of fresh cilantro leaves

Heat a grill pan until it is very hot. Drizzle the lime juice onto the steak, sprinkle with sugar, and season with salt and Szechuan pepper. Sear steak for 2 to 4 minutes on each side until cooked to your liking,* turning frequently and watching that it doesn't burn (the sugar will caramelize, but will also threaten to char). Rest for 10 minutes. Meanwhile, combine dressing ingredients and assemble salad. Slice steak thinly, place decoratively on salad, and serve with plenty of the tangy Thai dressing.

* Guide for cooking steak: for rare meat, sear for 1 minute for approximately ½ inch of thickness

---

Vegetables

Goan Eggplant Curry
173 calories per portion (250 with brown basmati rice)
Serves 2

- 1 teaspoon cumin seeds, dry roasted in a small frying pan
- 2 teaspoons coriander seeds, dry roasted in a small frying pan
- ½ teaspoon cayenne pepper
- ½ teaspoon ground turmeric
- 1 green chili pepper, seeded and finely sliced

2 garlic cloves, crushed

1 teaspoon grated fresh ginger

7 ounces water

10 ounces low-fat coconut milk

1 tablespoon tamarind paste

1 large eggplant, cut lengthwise into ¼-thick slices

Salt and pepper

Crush roasted cumin and coriander seeds in a mortar and pestle. Place in a large saucepan along with the cayenne, turmeric, chili, garlic, ginger, and the water. Bring to a simmer, then add the coconut milk and tamarind paste. Cook on a low heat for 10 minutes, stirring occasionally, until slightly thickened. Heat grill to medium high. Place eggplant on a foil-lined baking sheet and brush with a little of the curried sauce. Grill until they are soft and cooked through, turning once and brushing the other side with the sauce, 10 to 15 minutes. Place eggplant in a serving dish, and spoon on the rest of the hot curry sauce. If you want rice with your curry, include ⅓ cup cooked brown basmati rice per person. It's a decent Fast Day source of slow-release carbohydrates, and is nutty and nutrient-rich (+77 calories).

Butternut Ratatouille
148 calories per portion
Serves 4

A twist on the classic ratatouille—the butternut squash brings a new texture and color to the dish. I'd be inclined to eat it with a spoon.

> 10 ounces butternut squash, peeled, seeded, and cut
> into 1-inch chunks
> 2 tablespoons olive oil
> 1 teaspoon cumin seeds
> Salt and pepper
> Cooking spray
> 1 onion, finely chopped
> 1 eggplant, cut into ¾-inch cubes
> 1 tablespoon tomato paste
> 1 (14-ounce) can diced tomatoes
> 2 garlic cloves, crushed
> 7 ounces spinach leaves
> Fresh basil leaves and 1 tablespoon grated
> Parmesan to serve

Preheat oven to 400°F. Place butternut squash in a small roasting pan with the olive oil. Add cumin seeds, season well, and toss to coat. Bake for 20 minutes until tender, stirring halfway through cooking time. Spray a pan with cooking oil, sauté the onion until softened, add eggplant, and cook until lightly browned and cooked through. Add tomato paste, diced tomatoes, garlic, and roasted butternut squash. Season. Stir, cover, and cook for 10 to 15 minutes, until thickened and really savory. Add spinach for final 2 minutes of cooking time, sprinkle with torn basil and grated Parmesan, and serve.

Red Vegetables
164 calories per portion
Serves 4

2 tablespoons olive oil
3 red onions, each cut into 8 wedges
3 garlic cloves, crushed
4 carrots, peeled and cut into ½-inch chunks
2 beets, peeled and cut into ½-inch chunks
10.5 ounces sweet potato or pumpkin, peeled, seeded, and cut into ¾-inch chunks
1 head of radicchio or red chicory, quartered
Juice of half a lemon
2 sprigs fresh thyme
1 teaspoon honey
2 to 3 tablespoons water
Handful of fresh basil

In a heavy-bottomed pan, heat the oil, then add the vegetables, lemon juice, thyme, honey and water and stir well. Cover, bring to a simmer, and braise gently until the vegetables start to soften, 25 to 30 minutes, stirring occasionally to release any stickiness from the pan base. If it gets too dry, add another tablespoon of water. Season well and serve with torn basil leaves.

Sesame Tofu with Stir-Fry Snow Peas

345 calories per portion
Serves 1

Tofu needs a punch of flavor to drag it from insipidity: here, the beloved ginger-chili-lime trio does the business.

- 1 teaspoon soy sauce
- 1 teaspoon chili sauce
- 3.5 ounces firm tofu, cut into cubes, dried on paper towels
- 1 tablespoon sesame seeds
- 1 tablespoon peanut oil
- 1 leek, washed and finely sliced
- ¾-inch fresh ginger root, peeled and julienned
- 1 small zucchini, julienned
- 3.5 ounces snow peas, blanched for a minute in boiling water and rinsed with cold
- Juice of a lime
- Cilantro leaves to serve

Mix soy and chili sauces in a bowl and add tofu. Leave to marinate in the fridge for 1 hour, then coat them with sesame seeds. Heat a little oil in a nonstick frying pan and fry tofu for 2 minutes until golden, turning occasionally and very gently. Remove tofu from the pan and rest on paper towels. Put the remaining oil in the pan, add the leek and ginger, with any remaining marinade, and stir-fry until softened. Add zucchini, cook for another 2 minutes, then add snow peas. Serve vegetables topped with cubes of tofu. Sprinkle with cilantro and more sesame seeds.

Salads

Watermelon Salad with Feta and Black Pepper
214 calories per portion
Serves 4

And now for something completely different . . . We all know how to throw together a salad, but sometimes unusual ingredients can make a fine marriage. This quick combo uses watermelon, which is full of vitamins and, despite its sweetness, has a low GL thanks to its high water content. With feta and fresh pepper, the salad is a real summer sensation. Try it and see.

For the dressing
1 tablespoon balsamic vinegar
2 teaspoons Dijon mustard
1 garlic clove, crushed
1 tablespoon good olive oil

For the salad
2 pounds watermelon, cubed
7 ounces low-fat feta cheese, crumbled

1 red onion, thinly sliced
Handful fresh mint leaves, coarsely chopped
Freshly ground black pepper
Sea salt

Combine dressing ingredients. Assemble salad, toss with dressing, and serve.

Zucchini, Pea, and Ricotta Salad
181 calories per portion
Serves 4

For the dressing
Zest and juice of a lemon
2 tablespoons extra-virgin olive oil
1 teaspoon honey
Salt and pepper

4 young zucchini, peeled into ribbons
3.5 ounces just-cooked fresh or frozen peas
3.5 ounces pea shoots
7 ounces ricotta cheese

Combine dressing ingredients, assemble salad and dot with teaspoons of ricotta. Drizzle with the dressing and serve.

Carrot, Spinach, and Coconut Salad with Hot Grilled Halloumi

254 calories per portion
Serves 2

Olive oil cooking spray
3.5 ounces reduced-fat halloumi, sliced
Salt and pepper
For the salad
1 bag baby spinach leaves, coarsely chopped
2 carrots, peeled and grated
4 tablespoons grated fresh coconut

For the dressing
1 tablespoon olive oil
1 teaspoon black mustard or caraway seeds
Juice of a lime
Juice of an orange
Salt and pepper

Spray halloumi slices with a little olive oil, season, and sear in a hot grill pan for 30 seconds on each side. Serve the dressed salad piled on a plate with the hot halloumi on top.

Pen's Beet Salad
159 calories per portion
Serves 4

My friend Pen swears by the mystic power of her shredded beet salad. It may sound a bit low-key, but try it: it's truly a sublime mouthful . . .

For the salad
3 medium fresh beets, scrubbed, and coarsely grated
3 carrots, peeled and grated
1 small celery root, peeled and grated
1 green apple, grated

For the dressing
2 tablespoons horseradish sauce
2 tablespoons olive oil
1 tablespoon freshly squeezed lemon or orange juice
1 teaspoon spicy yellow mustard
1 garlic clove, crushed
Salt and pepper
1 tablespoon sesame or pumpkin seeds to serve

Toss the grated veggies with the dressing, top with seeds, and serve.

Soups

Tuscan Summer Bean Soup
178 calories per portion
Serves 4

1 tablespoon olive oil
1 onion, finely diced
2 celery stalks, finely diced
1 red bell pepper, seeded and finely diced
1 carrot, peeled and finely diced
2 garlic cloves, crushed
2 sprigs fresh thyme, leaves only
2 sprigs fresh rosemary
1 bay leaf
1 teaspoon smoked paprika
1 (14-ounce) can diced tomatoes
4 cups good vegetable broth
1 vegetable bouillon cube
Pinch of superfine sugar
1 (14-ounce) can cannellini beans, rinsed and drained
1 (14-ounce) can flageolet beans, rinsed and drained
3.5 ounces fava beans, shelled
3.5 ounces baby peas
Salt and pepper

In a large saucepan, heat the oil and add the onion and celery. Sauté until softened, then add the bell pepper, carrot, garlic, herbs, and paprika. Cook, stirring, for 3 to 4 minutes, or until the carrots and peppers begin to soften. Add the tomatoes, broth, bouillon cube, and sugar to bring out the flavor of the tomatoes. Bring to a simmer, then add the canned beans. Stir gently and simmer for 15 to 20 minutes; in the final 2 minutes of cooking time, add the fava beans and peas. Bring back to a simmer, season, and serve piping hot.

Super-Simple Fridge Gazpacho
113 calories per portion
Serves 2

This is as fine a summer soup as you could imagine. It matters that the tomatoes are ripe and flavorful. It matters that you eat this fresh from the fridge. After that, nothing else matters at all.

1 red bell pepper, seeded and coarsely chopped
10.5 ounces red tomatoes, ideally a mix of varieties
½ cucumber (5 to 7 ounces), coarsely chopped
1 red chili pepper, seeded and coarsely chopped
1 garlic clove
2 green onions, sliced
2 tablespoons red wine vinegar
1 tablespoon good olive oil
Salt and pepper
Six ice cubes (optional)

Puree all the vegetables—raw—in a food processor until smooth. Add vinegar, oil, ice, salt, and pepper and quickly blitz again. Serve cold—with ice cubes floating in it if you wish—with more finely diced cucumber, tomato, and green onion. Gazpacho does not freeze well, so make it on the day and serve fresh.

Vietnamese Shrimp Pho
48 calories per portion (add 10 to 15 calories for every 1.7 ounces of additional vegetable)
Serves 4

Pho is the way to go if you want a big bolt of flavor for very few calories. Add spring vegetables of your choosing—snow peas, sugar snap peas, shredded cabbage, ribboned carrots, green beans, shiitake mushrooms, or baby sweetcorn . . . As with all soups, the dish hinges on a good broth.

- 2 lemongrass stalks, outer leaves removed, finely chopped
- 2 teaspoons grated fresh ginger
- 4 kaffir lime leaves, torn
- 6 cups good vegetable broth
- 1 teaspoon palm sugar or light soft brown sugar
- 3 tablespoons Thai fish sauce
- Juice of a lime
- 8 jumbo shrimp, shelled and deveined
- 1.7 ounces bean sprouts

Fresh Thai basil leaves, mint, cilantro, and thinly sliced red chili pepper to serve

Use a mortar and pestle to grind the lemongrass, ginger, and kaffir lime leaves. Put the paste in a large saucepan with stock and boil for 10 minutes. Add sugar, fish sauce, and lime juice, tasting to check for balance. Cook shrimp in broth until they are pink, 2 to 3 minutes. Add bean sprouts, plenty of herbs, and red chili pepper to serve. You can also add shirataki noodles at negligible calorie cost: cook according to package directions, and ladle the piping hot pho on top.

Don't even think about it . . .

I included some of these "Straight to the Plate" ideas in *FastCook*, and they proved a popular way to get through dinner on a Fast Day with minimum fuss. Not recipes so much as great flavor combinations, these trios can be grabbed from your fridge and kitchen cupboards on days when you just don't want to think too hard about food. Use lemon juice, balsamic vinegar (I like it in spray form), or the basic Fast Day dressing (below) where necessary. Then just add a plate, a fork, and an appetite.

- Shredded white cabbage + sliced red onion + hard-boiled egg (1 medium), **100 calories**
- Smoked salmon (1.7 ounces) + hard-boiled egg (1 medium) + sliced fennel, **180 calories**

- Fava beans (3.5 ounces) + radicchio + pecorino (1 ounce), **196 calories**
- Lean roast beef (3.5 ounces) + horseradish crème fraîche (1 tablespoon) + romaine hearts, **203 calories**
- Chicken tikka pieces (4.5 ounces) + sliced beef tomato + cucumber raita (2 tablespoons), **216 calories**
- Avocado (half) + shrimp (5 ounces) + low-fat crème fraîche (1 tablespoon), **217 calories**
- Prosciutto (4 slices) + melon + strawberries, **228 calories**
- Mozzarella (1.7 ounces) + avocado (half) + 2 ripe tomatoes, **237 calories**
- Baby spinach + prosciutto (4 slices) + Parmesan (1 ounce), **244 calories**
- Low-fat hummus (3.5 ounces) + raw veggies + jalapeños, **246 calories**
- Canned tuna (3.5 ounces) + cannellini beans (3.5 ounces) + red onion, **268 calories**
- Cooked turkey breast (7 ounces) + arugula + pine nuts (2 teaspoons), **269 calories**
- Smoked chicken (5 ounces) + romaine lettuce + cashews (2 tablespoons), **276 calories**
- Blanched green beans + cooked jumbo shrimp (5 ounces) + low-fat feta (3.5 ounces), **289 calories**
- Roast beet (3.5 ounces) + low-fat halloumi (3.5 ounces) + arugula, **293 calories**
- Low-fat feta (3.5 ounces) + hard-boiled egg (1 medium) + red cabbage, **295 calories**
- Sardines in olive oil (3.5 ounces) + 10 cherry tomatoes + steamed broccoli florets, **323 calories**
- Smoked salmon (3.5 ounces) + watercress + 4 plum tomatoes, **354 calories**

- Beef carpaccio (5 ounces) + toasted pine nuts (2 teaspoons) + arugula + Parmesan (1 ounce), **404 calories**

The Fast Day Dressing
112 calories per tablespoon

1 tablespoon lemon juice
1 tablespoon white wine vinegar
2 tablespoons extra-virgin olive oil
2 teaspoons Dijon mustard
1 garlic clove, peeled and left whole
Salt and pepper

Whisk ingredients together and keep in an airtight jar in the fridge. It will last for a week. Remove garlic clove before eating.

Fast Day Snacks
As I have pointed out elsewhere, there's little point in grazing on a Fast Day. But some people need a little lift, particularly in the early days when their appetite is adjusting to the new routine. It's best to avoid easy carbs and go instead for fresh, raw ingredients. Have them prepped and handy in the fridge. Nuts, though high in calories, are full of protein and good fats, and just a few will help you feel full.

- Licorice to chew, **0 calories**
- 2 ounces cherries, **23 calories**
- 3.5 ounces blackberries, **25 calories**
- Fresh strawberries, **30 calories for 10**
- A miso soup packet, **32 calories**
- Crudités: carrot sticks, celery sticks, cucumber sticks, raw pepper, watercress, radishes, cherry tomatoes, approximately **40 calories** per serving
- 1 tablespoon cottage cheese, **40 calories**
- Apple slices, including skin and core—add a squeeze of lemon juice, **48 calories**
- 1 tablespoon hummus, **56 calories**
- A handful of frozen grapes, **60 calories**
- Pistachios, **60 calories for 10**
- Almonds, **80 calories for 6**
- 2 ounces plain edamame—steamed and served warm with a little salt, **84 calories**
- 1 ounce Edam, **85 calories**
- 1 hard-boiled egg, **90 calories** (depending on size)
- 1 tablespoon pumpkin and sunflower seeds, **90 calories**
- 3 cups air-popped popcorn, **148 calories**

FAST DAY COOKING TIPS IN A NUTSHELL

- Feel free to top up the leafy, low-calorie, low-GI vegetables beyond the quantities given in any recipe. It is difficult to pig out on leafy vegetables, and if you need volume, that's where you should get it.

- Some vegetables benefit from cooking, others are best eaten raw. Cooking certain vegetables—including carrots, spinach, mushrooms, asparagus, cabbage, and peppers—means you are breaking down the cell structure without destroying vitamins, allowing you to absorb more goodness.
- Fast Days should be low in fat, rather than no fat. A teaspoon of olive oil can be used in cooking or drizzled over vegetables for flavor, or use a cooking spray to get a thin film. Include a little oil dressing on your salads; it means that you are more likely to absorb their fat-soluble vitamins.
- The vitamin C in lemon or orange dressings helps the body to absorb more iron from leafy greens such as spinach and kale. Watercress with orange, for instance, is a great combination.
- Cook with a nonstick pan to cut down on calorie-dense fats. Add a splash of water if the food sticks. In summer, bring out the barbecue.
- Choose lower-fat cheeses and low-fat or skim milk.
- Similarly, avoid starchy white carbohydrates (bread, sticky rice, pasta) and opt instead for low-GI carbs such as legumes and slow-burn cereals. Choose brown rice and quinoa.
- Ensure that you get plenty of fiber on a Fast Day: eat the skin of apples and pears, have oatmeal for breakfast, keep those leafy vegetables coming in.
- Add flavor where you can: red pepper flakes will give a kick to any savory dish. Vinegars, including balsamic, will lend acidity. Add fresh herbs too—

they are virtually calorie free, but give personality to a plate.

- Eating some protein will help keep you full longer. Stick to the lean proteins, including vegetable protein from nuts and legumes. Remove the skin and fat from meat before eating.
- Use agave as a sweetener if required; it's low GI.

The FBD Shopping List: What to Have on Hand

Get in the habit of having Fast-friendly food around—just enough to allow you to grab a quick meal when you're fasting and famished.

In the Fridge

Eggs
Mackerel fillets
Smoked salmon
Low-fat hummus, low-fat plain yogurt, and crème fraîche
Feta, cottage cheese, and low-fat mozzarella
Green onions
Chili peppers
Fresh herbs
Nonstarchy veggies: cauliflower, broccoli, peppers, radishes, cherry tomatoes, celery, cucumber, mushrooms, lettuce, sugar snap peas, snow peas, salad, and spinach
Carrots
Lemons
Strawberries, blueberries, apples

In the Pantry

Canned tuna
Cans of beans and chickpeas
Cans of diced tomatoes
Tomato paste
Garlic
Onions (red and white)
Mustard (Dijon and spicy yellow)
Vinegar (balsamic and white wine; try balsamic spritzer on
   salad)
Olive oil
Cooking spray
Spices, including cumin and coriander
Red pepper flakes
Nuts (unsalted are preferable)
Pickles (guindillas, jalapeños, cornichons, capers)
Bouillon cubes and miso paste
Sea salt and freshly ground black pepper
Unsweetened muesli
Sugar-free jelly
Shirataki noodles
Miso soup packets

In the Freezer

Ginger root—it is best grated from frozen
Broth, in empty (clean) soup and milk cartons
Soup—homemade or store-bought, in single portions
Blueberries, a cool little snack (strawberries don't
   freeze well)

Six-Week Meal Plan, Under 500 Calories —Breakfast and Dinner

(for the recipes, see pages 103–137)

WEEK 1	BREAKFAST 100–250 calories	DINNER 200–350 calories
FAST DAY 1	Poached eggs (180 calories)	Goan eggplant curry and brown basmati rice (250 calories)
FAST DAY 2	Muesli, yogurt, and fruit (245 calories)	Lime and herb chicken salad (195 calories)

WEEK 2	BREAKFAST	DINNER
FAST DAY 1	Oat berry smoothie (220 calories)	Italian seafood salad (261 calories)
FAST DAY 2	2 boiled eggs, asparagus (180 calories)	Gazpacho (113 calories) and zucchini, pea, and ricotta salad (181 calories)

WEEK 3	BREAKFAST	DINNER
FAST DAY 1	Scrambled eggs (220 calories)	Goan eggplant curry (173 calories)
FAST DAY 2	Date and apricot smoothie (280 calories)	Lime and herb chicken salad (195 calories)

WEEK 4	BREAKFAST 150–250 calories	DINNER 300–350 calories
FAST DAY 1	Herring and mushrooms* (234 calories)	Watermelon and feta salad (214 calories)
FAST DAY 2	Poached egg and ham (170 calories)	Sticky salmon with ginger (335 calories)

WEEK 5	BREAKFAST	DINNER
FAST DAY 1	Scrambled eggs, shrimp, and cilantro (356 calories)	Carrot, spinach, and coconut salad with halloumi (254 calories)
FAST DAY 2	Yogurt, berries, almonds* (264 calories)	Tuscan bean soup (178 calories)

WEEK 6	BREAKFAST	DINNER
FAST DAY 1	Tricolore omelet (184 calories)	Chicken and mango salad (418 calories)
FAST DAY 2	Oat smoothie with apple, cinnamon, and vanilla (282 calories)	Butternut ratatouille (148 calories)

* See FastDiet Recipe book

143

Six Week Meal Plan, Under 600 Calories—
Dinner Only

WEEK 1	DINNER
FAST DAY 1	Spiced chicken with lentils and garlic (399 calories), served with green salad and Fast Day dressing
FAST DAY 2	Goan eggplant curry and brown basmati rice (250 calories), served with a store-bought whole grain naan (180 calories)

WEEK 2	
FAST DAY 1	Pho (48 calories), followed by Thai beef salad (351 calories)
FAST DAY 2	Tuscan bean soup (178 calories), followed by sticky salmon with ginger (335 calories)

WEEK 3	
FAST DAY 1	Butternut ratatouille (148 calories) with grilled chicken breast (127 calories), green salad and Fast Day dressing
FAST DAY 2	Gazpacho (113 calories), followed by sesame tofu and snow pea stir-fry (345 calories)

WEEK 4	DINNER
FAST DAY 1	Deb's monkfish with roasted peppers/tomatoes (289 calories), served with brown basmati rice (77 calories) and green beans (20–30 calories)
FAST DAY 2	Miso soup (32 calories), followed by sirloin steak (183 calories) with red vegetables (164 calories) and broccolini (40 calories)

WEEK 5	
FAST DAY 1	Chicken and mango salad (418 calories)
FAST DAY 2	Tricolore omelet (184 calories), followed by Italian seafood salad (261 calories)

WEEK 6	
FAST DAY 1	Salmon tartare (282 calories) with zucchini, pea, and ricotta salad (181 calories)
FAST DAY 2	Shrimp on toast (310 calories), followed by lime and herb chicken salad (195 calories)

Chapter 8

Sticking with It in the Weeks Ahead

So, you've absorbed the new boot camp method for the FastBeach Diet. You're energized and raring to go. But what happens in week three and a bit, when you might need a boost? That's the time to turn to friends, and to take yourself aside for a stern talking to. Here are practical ways to help yourself out of the rough and into the sunlit uplands of Intermittent Fasting . . .

Buddy Up

A supportive friend may well be one of your greatest assets in the weeks ahead; you might find that they join in, and you'll develop a network of common experience.

Since the plan appeals to men and women equally, couples report that they find it more manageable to do it together (as the testimonials in chapter 9 demonstrate); not only are there anecdotes and experiences to share, but meal times are made infinitely easier if you're eating with someone who understands the rudiments of the plot. It's remarkable how reassuring it is to know that you're not alone.

Go to the Forum

What's particularly interesting to me is that the FastDiet has developed into such a lively conversation. Neither Michael nor I are interested in promoting diet dependency, only in investigating an idea that seems to have truly life-changing potential. Over the past year, that conversation has been evolving and growing online. To tune in to the discussion, and to discover countless tips and takes to make the Fast Diet work for you, go to www.thefastdiet.co.uk. Or check out the many Facebook groups—ours is at www.facebook .com/thefastdiet.co.uk.

Fast Thinking: Some Final Words to Get Your Brain on Board

Hold Yourself in High Esteem

At the risk of sounding like a fridge magnet, here are some of my favorite words from the Buddha which may help to ground and inspire you in the weeks ahead: "You can search throughout the entire universe for someone who is more deserving of your love and affection than you are yourself, and that person is not to be found anywhere. You yourself, as much as anybody in the entire universe, deserve your love and affection."

"Do or Do Not. There is No Try."

These words, from Yoda (another favorite), are infinitely wise and work just as well when tackling weight loss as they do in the swamps of Dagobah when contemplating a broken X-wing fighter. The point is to get on with it. No excuses. No attempts. But action. Now. As someone somewhere once said: just do it. Go into the next six weeks with your head, and your aspirations, high. But remain playful. So you missed a meal? So what. Just keep going.

Don't Give Up, You're Already Partway There

Having a period in your day when food simply isn't allowed to pass your lips achieves many things, both physiological and psychological. It is galvanizing. It can be liberating. It certainly prevents random snacking, and it might also alert you to how often you do this in the normal course of events. Use your success on a Fast Day to inform your actions on a non-Fast Day. Simply realizing that you can curb your appetite and cope with a bit of hunger is a great start. You are already on the right road.

Customize

The key—whether you're doing the FastDiet or the souped-up six-week FastBeach Diet—is to find a plan that works for you, which means you may need to experiment a little until you find your best fit. Once you've completed the six-week FastBeach Diet, your aim is to arrive at a sustainable, lifelong plan. So relax a little and return to the classic 5:2 FastDiet. In fact, rather than think of 5:2 as "a diet," which in its modern usage is loaded with quick-fix connotations, perhaps begin to see it as stemming from the classical Greek *"diaita."* This roughly translates as "a manner of living." A way of life. A commitment to health and well-being. As I hope you'll have gathered, there are no promises here, just proposals. Think of them as proposals for a longer, stronger life.

Be Sensible, and If It Feels Wrong, Stop

It's vital that this strategy—both the original 5:2 format and the turbo version—should be practiced in a way that's flexible and forgiving. Take each day as it comes. It's OK to break the rules if you need to. If you're concerned about any aspect of IF, see your doctor.

Be Kind to Yourself

Try not to associate fasting with discomfort; be gentle to cultivate the changes you desire and deserve; don't dwell on the downside, for instance, if a Fast Day is broken. It's no biggie. Move along. Do, however, congratulate yourself, reinforcing the positive feedback loop which, as we saw in chapter 4, really helps when you're trying to break and make habits. Every completed Fast Day means potential weight loss and quantifiable health gain. You're already winning.

As my other guru and fellow Brightonian, Fatboy Slim, famously sang:

We've come a long, long way together,
Through the hard times and the good,
I have to celebrate you, baby,
I have to praise you like I should.

Dead right. Make this your shower song for the next six weeks.

Reward Yourself . . .

With shoes, not booze; put the money you save toward . . . well, how about a new swimsuit? But which one? First, a few friendly tips for women dieters out there . . .

One Piece, Madam, or Two?

Getting near naked in front of strangers (or worse, friends) is one of the great hurdles in a woman's fashion life, whatever her age. So what to wear on that beach once you've completed your FastBeach Diet and it's time for the great reveal? As a fashion editor, I spent a chunk of my career deliberating on such things in newspapers and magazines, and *The FastBeach Diet* seems the obvious place to share a few of my favorite beachside tricks.

While a one-piece swimsuit gives a sinuous, continuous line, it can also look a bit old-fashioned, as if you're en route to the public swimming baths with a rubber cap, goggles, and protective footwear. Dare to fling on a bikini (even if you haven't done so in years), and I promise, you'll feel immediately racy—off to the Hamptons or St. Tropez, the wind in your hair and the world at your sandy feet. Get it right and there are three things to love about a bikini: va, va, and voom.

According to fashion lore, a bikini is not a bikini unless it can be pulled through a wedding ring—which means that in its meager embrace, there's nowhere to hide. A truly great bikini (and you might only ever meet one in a lifetime) can, however, perform untold magic. Here's how to track yours down . . .

Size

Sounds basic, but do ensure that your bikini is the right size. Always try before you buy; that's what the plastic cover is there for.

Shape

If you want your bikini to work, rather than simply loaf about on a lounge chair, look for the following:

• Underwiring, which will stop your chest heading south

• A top with clip fastenings, not ties: these will give you added stability and enhance your shape

• A tie-side bottom, though, is adjustable and therefore more forgiving than the set-side bikini pants which tend to bite into your behind like a hungry shark

• High-leg bikini bottoms will elongate a leg, but can be demanding; try before you buy, so you arrive at a cut which suits your butt

• As a 46-year-old mother of two, I prefer a bikini bottom that has a slightly higher waistband; that extra half inch of fabric serves to contain a bit of a tummy

- But, counterintuitive as it may seem, your bottom will appear smaller if you house it in a little less fabric. I'm not suggesting that you go for the Brazilian "floss" bikini, just something that doesn't completely cover every scrap of flesh as if you've had your butt wallpapered.

- A big bust will benefit from a halter top—chiefly because it offers maximum support; you get a great cleavage as an added bonus.

- By contrast, bandeaus only really work on flatter chests; on more ample busts, you'll get a curious eruptive effect, like brioche on the rise.

Color

Fashion editors know as a matter of lore that particular colors complement certain skin tones.

- Red is very demanding on almost everyone—leave it to *Baywatch*.

- Acid yellow is tricky for pale skin.

- The aquas are brilliant for most complexions, with the plus that you'll complement the sea.

- Neons are cool, but suit a darker skin tone best. They're also very grabby on the eye, so you'll need buckets of body confidence to pull them off.

- White is infinitely more challenging than black. Always.

- Chocolate brown is perennially chic; khaki is kind; navy is no-nonsense and benevolent, like a nanny, and a softer alternative to black.

- I like a subtle animal print—something faded in the taupe/stone/beige color range, not the kind of aggressive print that looks as if it's on the attack.

- Polka dots are fun in the sun, but can be infantilizing, so wear with caution, or plenty of chutzpah.

THE TANNING TRICK

A little lick of sun exposure is no bad thing (it is thought to combat depression and aid sleep); what's more, by some fabulous trick of the light, a tan will lend tone and shave off pounds. Just don't overdo it. Use the correct UVA and UVB protection, avoid tanning beds, and, if in doubt, use a self-tanning product—exfoliating first to avoid those tell tale Tigger stripes.

TRY THIS FOR THIGHS: A WORD ON CELLULITE

So many products, so little use . . . I'm not sure that lasers, vacuum massage, micro-encapsulated caffeine tights, infrared light, retinol serum infusions or radio-frequency treatments will do anything much to help banish the orange peel. So, what might? All of the following are recommended as ways to help combat cellulite. The good news? On the FastBeach Diet, you'll be doing most of them already:

- Eat more plants and whole grains.
- Cut out processed food.
- Drink plenty of water.
- Cut back on salt.
- Take regular exercise.
- Get your circulation going: perhaps try body-brushing and lymphatic drainage massage; the jury's out on how effective they are as anti-cellulite treatments. But they can't hurt, and can feel great.

And, Last But by No Means Least . . .

Some handy advice for men. Your choice of swimwear depends largely on how much you want to reveal and how much you choose to conceal as you stroll from turf to surf.

Speedos

If you are an exceptionally good swimmer, or built like Tom Daley, then Speedos are clearly your beachtime buddy. They are, however, quite unforgiving, leaving very little to the imagination (Stella McCartney joked that Daley's minuscule trunks were the hardest part of the Great Britain's Olympics uniforms to design because there was no room for the pattern). In their favor, briefs let you swim with ease, dry almost immediately, and ensure that you don't take your keys, wallet, and phone swimming by mistake. They're also increasingly popular; if you're into manscaping and not averse to strutting your stuff, then do feel free.

A bold swirling pattern can easily go a bit Rod Stewart— so look for block color, with a comfortable mesh inner lining. If, once you've given them a whirl (and, as with all swimwear, do try before you buy), you look less like David Gandy and more Ray Winstone in *Sexy Beast*, perhaps spring for a little more cover.

Trunks

The fitted boxer trunk has been a beachside hit since 2006, when Daniel Craig emerged from the sea in *Casino Royale* wearing his baby-blue Grigioperla minishorts. Sales in smaller shorts have been on the rise ever since: according to the bodywear buyer at Selfridges, "everyone's moving down a shape—boxer short–wearers are moving into trunks, and trunks to briefs. Young, body-conscious men are getting the confidence to wear smaller shapes." If you're in the market for trunks, look for a retro sports style—Orlebar Brown leads the market here (think Jude Law in *The Talented Mr. Ripley*); navy is the best-selling color at Marks & Spencer in the UK—chiefly because it is unerringly chic without being unduly attention seeking.

Board Shorts

Popular as they may be, board shorts are hardly the most practical option—the beach equivalent of wearing jeans at the gym. But board shorts are cool, and refreshingly modest. If you can cope with the drag through the water, and don't mind surfer-dude graphics and a tan line that stops at your knees, they're hot. Try Vilebrequin for that suave French Riviera feel. If you can actually stand up on a surfboard, then look for Australian brands such as Rip Curl and Billabong, which have got the technical details (stretch fabric, seam reduction, ergonomic cut, quick-dry material, Velcro pockets) just right.

Chapter 9

Fast Talk: Encouragement from FastDiet Fans

Tanya, 41, Berkshire, UK
76 pounds lost in a year
"At my heaviest, I weighed 244 pounds! I was so big; I couldn't see how I could ever return to a healthy weight. I'd tried other diets and hated the feelings of guilt when I ate something 'naughty.' I used to give up and eat more. It was a vicious circle.

"Then, I heard about the 5:2 diet and on January 7, 2013, I started Intermittent Fasting. Initially I did a combination of 5:2 and some weeks 4:3. As the weight came off, the better I felt about myself and the more energy I had. I started walking with a friend on the days I was fasting. This kept me motivated; I used to visualize the differences to my appearance and also the health changes taking place within my body. I've heard that to break a habit (in my case eating) you need to replace it with another habit; mine became fasting.

"I now weigh around 168 pounds. That's another thing that's changed; I'm less obsessed with the scales and more interested in how I feel and how my clothes look on my changed body. I have taken the control back over what I eat and when. I understand my body more, know that I have made a massive difference to my health and feel absolutely fantastic!"

Louise Davey, 47, Australia
13 pounds lost in 10 months

"I have lost 13 pounds doing 5:2 since April last year. I heard an interview on the radio, downloaded the documentary, went and bought the book. The rest is history. Thanks, Michael. I will be doing this for life now. At first it was to lose some weight, but having watched the documentary online, my main reason for doing the Intermittent Fasting is mental/brain health. Coming from a family with Alzheimer's, I do not want to go down that road. This is good motivation in and of itself, but I do love a challenge. So, making interesting meals and working out how to get through a day is also quite fun. Along the way I have also found many others who do it and have convinced a lot of my friends that this is the way forward if you want to live a long and HEALTHY life."

Jeanne White, 42, San Francisco
10 pounds lost in 8 months

"Like many FastDieters before me, I'm sure, I fell into this diet, or rather, way of life, after reaching a point that nothing else I was doing was really making a difference. At 42, with two school-age boys, a husband, a home, and a full-time job, I felt like I was always on the go and didn't give much thought to calories. As a decades-long non-meat eater,

I felt I was 'healthy,' but gave little thought to the popcorn, chips, or goldfish crackers I'd snack on with my kids after school/work. After reading about the FastDiet and watching the subsequent interviews with Dr. Mosley, I thought I would give it a try. The first two days I chose, a Monday and a Wednesday, were difficult, I have to be honest! I recall being in the basement at work and looking at a stack of paper thinking, 'I'm just going to have to eat the paper.' But, I stuck through it, read everything I could find on the FastDiet, joined the Facebook page, etc., and came up with a meal plan that started working immediately.

"I've lost a total of about 10 pounds since June 2013, and I've continued with the program to maintain this healthy weight. Better yet, I feel great too, full of energy, able to last through rigorous yoga classes, and sleeping like a baby. I am an absolute creature of habit, and am quite content eating relatively similar things daily, so the FastDiet is easy for me to stick with, as I've found items that are easy to cook and that I genuinely enjoy."

Glory Puljak, 39, Australia
44 pounds lost in 8 months
"It's been 8 months now and I've lost 44 pounds! It just keeps falling off! This has never happened to me before. I have never been able to shift this much weight! I love it so much because I can still have my Friday night drinks and some dessert on the weekend and my social life doesn't suffer because of it. I feel so healthy, have so much energy and I feel so switched on. This, for me, is a life change that I will continue to do for ever! I cannot thank the FastDiet enough!

I also need to add that I walk or jog every day! This just helps me clear my mind and get my heart pumping."

Joan Rijkels, 67, The Hague, Netherlands
Over 42 pounds lost in 18 months
"In January 2012, I went to the doctor for a checkup and was told that I had an 18% chance of contracting a heart or vascular disease; at 20% they prescribe medication to lower cholesterol. My cholesterol level was 251 and I weighed 196 pounds. At 66 years old I decided to make a change to lead a healthier life.

"In August of 2012, I saw Michael Mosley's documentary on Intermittent Fasting. I started immediately. In January of 2013, I bought the book.

"Now it is January 2014, and I weigh 153.5 pounds. My cholesterol levels have dropped from 251 to 135 in two years. Also, I have arthritis and my BSE levels (blood sedimentation rate for erythrocytes) which never dropped below 6 for years, dropped to 2 after just six months on the diet.

"This diet has brought benefits to many people in my family: my sister's cholesterol hasn't been this low in 10 years. My other sister and her husband are both on the 5:2 for health benefits as opposed to weight loss, but she has lost 18–22 pounds, whilst her husband's cholesterol has dropped dramatically. My son-in-law had a triple bypass when he was 30 because of cholesterol problems and within five months of this diet has lost 33 pounds! My daughter has lost 22 pounds as well . . . the list goes on!

"Fasting feels great and I tell everyone that the reason it's sustainable is that if you don't manage to stick to 500 calories on one day . . . there's always tomorrow!"

Sandi Mueller, 70, Colorado
19 pounds lost in 10 weeks

"Your diet is the most amazing program I have ever been on. After 10 weeks, I have lost 19 pounds. More importantly, I feel terrific! I have had sinus problems and chronic bronchitis all my life. Now, my sinuses are clear and I can breathe freely. I am 70 years old and I have not felt this vibrant in decades. My 73-year-old husband has lost 20.8 pounds and I am certain that his cholesterol level has dropped. His cardiac specialist will be astounded. My sister, who told me about your diet, was able to reduce her prediabetic glucose level from 100 to 86 in five weeks. Our youngest daughter with irritable bowel syndrome has been symptom-free since her second week on your diet.

"Thank you for taking the time and effort to discover this revolutionary program. I call it the Fountain of Youth Diet. We all plan to continue this diet for the rest of our lives. You have brought health and hope to millions of people worldwide who could only look forward to a bleak future before your remarkable discovery."

Ruth Ellis, 45, Yorkshire, UK
Over 40 pounds lost in a year

"I chose the FastDiet for its potential long-term benefits. The fact that it also helps you lose weight was an added bonus. In 12 months I have lost 8 inches off my waist and more than 40 pounds in weight. My husband is doing the diet along with me and he has lost over 55 pounds.

"On Fast Days, stir-fries and Asian-style soups are our favored choice, with plenty of vegetables and some protein (chicken, lean meat, shrimp, squid, fish). Using spices, herbs, and garlic helps to boost the flavor and keep it interesting. I prefer to save most of my calories for the evening meal as I find that if I have something to eat earlier in the day it makes it harder to fight the cravings. I also sleep better if I've had a decent evening meal. If you find yourself feeling light-headed during a Fast Day it's often due to your sodium levels dropping, so a small pinch of salt often sorts that out. The morning after a fast I find it best to have either a protein-based or whole grain breakfast and not overload on the carbs. When I first started eating this way, I would often overcompensate and eat too much on the non-Fast Days, but over time this settled down and it has helped me to regulate my appetite on other days. I don't worry about calories on non-Fast Days, but I make wiser choices, rarely snack, don't overload my plate, and no longer have such a sweet tooth."

Susie White, late fifties, Northumberland, UK
Lost 2 inches around waist in 18 months
"At a yearly Well Woman checkup I was told my waist measurement put me just in the 'red' and that I should eat less and exercise more. The health warnings were there. I felt pretty down because I eat healthily anyway, garden almost every day and walk quite a lot. For a postmenopausal woman, it is very easy to feel depressed about putting on weight, especially round the middle. I felt it was a gradual process and that it was becoming very hard to reverse.

"The *Horizon* program came at just the right time; I was impressed by Michael Mosley's scientific approach, and decided the very next week to go for it. It's not so much the thought of living longer but the thought of living fitter and hopefully being a bit less likely to get diabetes or dementia.

"Initial weight loss made me feel so uplifted. There was an immediate feeling of having more energy and my brain feeling sharper. I've followed the FastDiet ever since, twice a week, except for one day a week over Christmas and New Year. I didn't have loads to lose and I'm very happy with losing 10 pounds. It's the reverse of the depressing downward spiral of putting on weight. Feeling fitter and leaner gives me the spirit to go on fasting. I'm not exaggerating if I describe the FastDiet as changing my life."

Kyra Challen, 25, Bedfordshire, UK
12 pounds lost in first 12 weeks
"When I decided I wanted to try the FastDiet, one of my main worries was that I would be sitting down to a simple dinner and my husband Chris would be there digging into pizza and chips, so I was surprised and relieved when he suggested we both follow the FastDiet together. This makes meals easier as we have the same thing, just like on non-Fast Days, and is also really good for my motivation and for sharing ideas about what works and what doesn't.

"We still manage our Fast Days differently during the day—he prefers to have breakfast and fast all day, whereas I prefer to fast from getting up until lunch, but come dinnertime we eat together. It is really helpful to know we are both going through the same temptations during the day and it definitely makes me think twice before 'cheating' on a Fast Day.

"Since starting the FastDiet, the main changes I have

noticed are not just around weight loss: I have more energy and my appetite every day, even non-Fast Days, has dramatically decreased; I just don't want to eat as much any more, which is going to be a life-saving habit, I think. By Christmas I had lost 12 pounds after following the diet for about 12 weeks and my husband lost 16 pounds in that same time, so our combined weight loss is almost 30 pounds. We both fit easily into clothes from a few years ago now!"

Carol Massey

"This diet enabled me in the first week to join in and socialize and still lose weight. I now want to lose my excess weight with three fasts per week. I don't feel daunted by this at all, that is a first. I am so enjoying planning my meals ahead of time. I love a stir-fry and the Fast Days energize me the next day. I am eating healthy food on non-Fast Days and don't feel tempted to overeat.

"It's true what the book says: 'my appetite has been retuned.' I see how I was eating when I didn't need food but was thirsty. I drink very weak Earl Grey tea all day and never feel hungry, except when it's time for my main meal. I grazed before and see why the weight kept coming back. I now just eat at mealtimes and take time to savor food. And knowing that if I really do want a piece of cake I can have it is great. Funnily, the urge for these foods has gone. I made a batch of ginger cookies the other day and had a couple, then gave the rest away to a grateful skinny friend! Because I know I have a 'choice' it changes everything. How great is that?"

Jeff Chinnock, mid-forties, Devon, UK
28 pounds lost in a year

"We have been doing the 5:2 diet since September 2012 after seeing the *Horizon* program. We have stuck to it ever since—apart from a brief Christmas break—and it has completely transformed how we eat, our relationship with food, as well as having a positive impact on our health and waistlines.

"My wife has recently been diagnosed with an endocrine disease that usually causes uncontrollable weight gain (and a risk of diabetes) and everyone has said that there is little you can do about this. But by doing the FastDiet she has managed to maintain and even lose some weight without affecting her nutrition, and she has avoided diabetes.

"At the same time, the book has helped to remind me of the original inspiration for adopting this way of eating (not sure I would describe it as a diet) and the tips and recipes have been extremely useful in helping us provide a bit more variety to what we eat. I have lost over 28 pounds and feel much healthier—the only downside being the need to buy new clothes . . ."

From the www.thefastdiet.co.uk forum:

Angie090465
"At first I worried like everyone else about fasting, would I get so hungry I would faint? Would I even last the day?

"The only way to find out was to actually go ahead and give this fasting way of life a try! I picked 2 days and I was pleasantly surprised to find that it wasn't as difficult as I had feared, and the more fasts I completed the easier it became . . . I did not lose weight straightaway, this is a common question from newbies, because when the pounds don't fall off right away they assume it does not work! But you have to give it time, at least a few weeks . . . I started losing a few pounds each month which I was happy about. I started at 139 pounds and wanted to lose at least 10 pounds and I didn't mind how long it would take as for me this would become a way of life.

"Now it's April 2014 and I am hovering around 131 or 132; I am happy with that and have now switched to 6:1, ie where you do one fast a week to maintain.

"I do hope my story inspires others to give 5:2 a go, I now enjoy the health benefits of it, my skin is so much clearer, I have much more energy, and I can get up at 6 a.m. in the morning without the lethargic feeling anymore!"

sylvestra

"I could say I've 'only' lost 1 pound this week . . . BUT I started doing 5:2 to kick-start my weight loss again after reaching a plateau. I've been doing 5:2 for three weeks and have lost FIVE pounds in that time—added to my other weight loss, since February I have lost 40 pounds in total— that's 20% of my original weight and I'm two-thirds of the way to my target weight. It may not continue like this every week but as long as the trend is downwards I'll be a happy bunny. The 5:2 certainly does make you rethink your eating. As I posted on another thread—I started using 'cauliflower rice' and 'zucchini spaghetti' on fast days as they're low on calories, low on carbs, and lighter on the digestion and now find I prefer this to the real thing which I'm finding dull!"

From Twitter:

@follielincoln
Started @TheFastDietBook 1yr ago & lost a stubborn 23lb. Wish the 20 yr old 5-stone heavier me knew what this 40-something does!

@TheFastDietBook
RT from double Olympian @NathanJDouglas 'the #fastdiet is the diet that I recommend to people when they ask my advice, it's a great diet'

@Mrs_Metters
#FastDiet 4 months, 32 fast days, 48000kcal not consumed, 17lb lost, 3 BMI points dropped, #SkinnyJeansOn

@JennieJHill
I've been doing this 4 weeks, have lost 4 kilos, and my bloke has lost 5. Also healthier. It's wonderful

@LucyKStirk
Thanks for your inspiration. Started in Sept and just passed the 3st lost mark! #doesnotfeellikeadiet

@Caffy49
I call it my Guiltless Diet, on my 5 days of normal eating I don't beat myself up if I have an indulgent day. Easy dieting

NOTES

1. Hamid R. Farschi, Moira A. Taylor, and Ian A. Macdonald, "Beneficial Metabolic Effects of Regular Meal Frequency on Dietary Thermogenesis, Insulin Sensitivity, and Fasting Lipid Profiles in Healthy Obese Women," *American Journal of Clinical Nutrition* 81, no. 2 (2005).
2. Krista A. Varady, et al., "Short-term Modified Alternate-Day Fasting: A Novel Dietary Strategy for Weight Loss and Cardioprotection in Obese Adults," *American Journal of Clinical Nutrition* 90, no. 5 (2009).
3. Andy Coghlan, "Our Liver Vacation: Is a Dry January Really Worth It?" *New Scientist* 2950 (January 13, 2014).
4. "Sainsbury's Wine Labels to Display Calorie Counts," *The Guardian*, February 20, 2014, http://www.theguardian.com/business/2014/feb/20/sainsburys-wine-label-calorie-counts.
5. Brian Wansink and Koert van Ittersum, "Shape of Glass and Amount of Alcohol Poured: Comparative Study of Effect of Practice and Concentration," *British Medical Journal* 331, no. 7531 (2005).
6. Susanne H. A. Holt, Janette C. Brand Miller, and Peter Petocz, "An Insulin Index of Foods: The Insulin Demand Generated by 1000-kJ Portions of Common Foods," *American Journal of Clinical Nutrition,* 66, no. 5 (1997).
7. Brian Wansink and Pierre Chandon, "Can 'Low-Fat' Nutrition Labels Lead to Obesity?" *Journal of Marketing Research,* 43, no. 4 (2006).
8. Paul J. Kenny, "Reward Mechanisms in Obesity: New Insights and Future Directions," *Neuron* 69, no. 4 (2011). *See also* Paul M. Johnson and Paul J. Kenny, "Dopamine D2 Receptors in Addiction-like Reward Dysfunction and Compulsive Eating in Obese Rats," *Nature Neuroscience,* 13, no. 5 (2010).
9. Barbara Rolls and Julie Flood, "Eating Soup Will Help Cut Calories at Meals," presented at the Experimental Biology Conference in Washington (May 2007).
10. Susan E. Berkow and Neal Barnard, "Vegetarian Diets and Weight Status," *Nutrition Reviews* 64, no. 4 (April 2006). *See also* M. Rosell, et al., "Weight Gain Over 5 Years in 21,966 Meat-eating, Fish-eating, Vegetarian, and Vegan Men and Women," *International Journal of Obesity* 30, no. 9 (2006).
11. Youfa Wang and May A. Beydoun, "Meat Consumption is Associated with Obesity and Central Obesity among US Adults," *International Journal of Obesity* 33, no. 6 (2009).
12. Bonnie Beezhold and Carol Johnston, "The Impact of Vitamin C Depletion on a Short-term Diet," reported at Experimental Biology presentation (San Francisco, 2006).
13. Susan Swithers and Terry L. Davidson, "A Pavlovian Approach to the Problem of Obesity," *International Journal of Obesity* 28 (July 2004). *See also*

Notes

Susan Swithers and Terry L. Davidson, "A Role for Sweet Taste: calorie predictive relations in energy regulation by rats," *Behavioral Neuroscience* 122 (February 2008).

14. Arthur Eumann Mesas, et al., "The Effect of Coffee on Blood Pressure and Cardiovascular Disease in Hypertensive Individuals," *American Journal of Clinical Nutrition* 94 (October 2011). *See also:* Susanna C. Larsson and Nicola Orsini, "Coffee Consumption and Risk of Stroke: A Dose-response Meta-analysis of Prospective Studies," *American Journal of Epidemiology* (September 2011); Anna Floegel, et al., "Coffee Consumption and Risk of Chronic Disease in the European Prospective Investigation into Cancer and Nutrition (EPIC)—German Study," *American Journal of Clinical Nutrition* (April 2012).

15. Francesco C. Cappuccio, et al., "Meta-analysis of Short Sleep Duration and Obesity in Children and Adults," *Sleep* 31, no. 5 (2008).

16. Shahrad Taheri, et al., "Short Sleep Duration is Associated with Reduced Leptin, Elevated Ghrelin, and Increased Body Mass Index," *PloS Medicine* (December 2004).

17. Shahrad Taheri, "The Interactions Between Sleep, Metabolism, and Obesity," *International Journal of Sleep and Wakefulness* 1 (2007).

18. Jean-Phillipe Chaput, et al., "Short Sleep Duration is Associated with Reduced Leptin Levels and Increased Adiposity: Results from the Québec Family Study," *Obesity* 15 (January 2007).

19. Brian Wansink and Matthew M. Cheney, "Super Bowls: Serving Bowl Size and Food Consumption," *Journal of the American Medical Association* 293, no. 14 (April 2005).

20. Paul Rozin, et al., "The Ecology of Eating: Smaller Portion Sizes in France than in the United States Help Explain the French Paradox," *Psychological Science* 14, no. 5 (September 2003).

21. Brian Wansink and Koert van Ittersum, "The Perils of Plate Size: Waist, Waste, and Wallet," *Journal of Marketing* (not yet published), available at www.smallplatemovement.org/doc/big_bowls.doc. *See also Brian Wansink and Koert van Ittersum*, "The Visual Illusions of Food: Why Plates, Bowls, and Spoons can Bias Consumption Volume, *The Journal of the Federation of American Societies for Experimental Biology* 20 (2006).

22. Jack F. Hollis, et al., "Weight Loss During the Intensive Intervention Phase of the Weight-Loss Maintenance Trial," *American Journal of Preventative Medicine* 35, no. 2 (August 2008).

23. Brian Wansink and Jeffery Sobal, "Mindless Eating: The 200 Daily Food Decisions We Overlook," *Environment and Behavior* 39, no. 1 (January 2007).

24. Brian Wansink, James E. Painter, and Yeon-Kyung Lee, "The Office Candy Dish: Proximity's Influence on Estimated and Actual Consumption," *International Journal of Obesity* 30 (May 2006).

25. Brian Wansink and Junyong Kim, "Bad Popcorn in Big Buckets: Portion Sizes can Influence Intake as Much as Taste," *Journal of Nutrition Education and Behavior* 37, no. 5 (2005). *See also* Brian Wansink, James E. Painter, and Jill North, "Bottomless Bowls: Why Visual Cues of Portion Size May Influence Intake," *Obesity Research* 13, no. 1 (2005).

26. Baba Shiv and Stephen M. Nowlis, "The Effect of Distractions While Tasting a Food Sample: The Interplay of Informational and Affective Components in Subsequent Choice," *Journal of Consumer Research* 31, no. 3 (December 2004).

27. Phillippa lally, et al., "How Are Habits Formed: Modelling Habit Formation in the Real World," *European Journal of Social Psychology* 40, no. 6 (October 2010).

28. Wendy Wood and David Thomas Neal, "Automatically in Situ: direct context cuing of habits in daily life," *The Psychology of Action, Volume 2: Mechanisms of Human Action,* (Oxford University Press: 2008).

29. Ayelet Fishbach, Tal Eyal, and Stacey R. Finkelstein, "How Positive and Negative Feedback Motivate Goal Pursuit," *Social and Personality Psychology Compass* 4, no. 8 (2010).

30. Caroline Davis, "From Passive Overeating to 'Food Addiction': A Spectrum of Compulsion and Severity," *Obesity* (April 2013).

31. Leigh Newman, "Life Changes: How to Create New Habits," *Huffington Post,* November 26, 2012, http://www.huffingtonpost.com/2012/11/26/life-changes-how-to-create-habits_n_1970105.html.

32. Michelle R. van Dellen and Rick H. Hoyle, "Regulatory Accessibility and Social Influences on State Self-Control," *Personality and Social Psychology Bulletin* 36, no. 2 (2010).

33. Karen Van Proeyen, et al., "Beneficial Metabolic Adaptations Due to Endurance Exercise Training in the Fasted State," *Journal of Applied Physiology* 110 (January 2011).

34. Maria Maraki, et al., "Acute Effects of a Single Exercise Class on Appetite, Energy Intake and Mood. Is there a time of day effect?" *Appetite* 45 (December 2005).

35. Karen Van Proeyen, et al., "Training in the Fasted State Improves Glucose Tolerance during Fat-Rich Diet," *Journal of Physiology* 588, pt. 21 (November 2010).

36. Steve Stannard, et al., "Adaptations to Skeletal Muscle with Endurance Exercise Training in the Acutely Fed Versus Overnight-Fasted State," *Journal of Science and Medicine in Sport* 13, no. 4 (July 2010).

37. Mehrdad Heydari, Judith Freund, and Stephen H. Boutcher, "The Effect of High-Intensity Intermittent Exercise on Body Composition of Overweight Young Males," *Journal of Obesity* 2012 (2012).

38. Martin J. Gibala, et al., "Physiological Adaptations to Low-Volume, High-Intensity Interval Training in Health and Disease," *The Journal of Physiology* 590, no. 5 (2012).

39. Neil A. King, et al., "Metabolic and Behavioral Compensatory Responses to Exercise Interventions: Barriers to Weight Loss," *Obesity* 15, no. 6 (2007).

40. Carolina Werle, Brian Wansink, and Collin Payne, "Just Thinking About Exercise Makes Me Serve More Food. Physical Activity and Calorie Compensation," *Appetite* 56, no. 2 (2010).

41. Richard S. Metcalfe, et al., "Towards the Minimal Amount of Exercise for Improving Metabolic Health: Beneficial Effects of Reduced-Exertion High-Intensity Interval Training," *European Journal of Applied Physiology* 112, no. 7 (2012).

42. Melanie S. Hood, et al, "Low-Volume Interval Training Improves Muscle Oxidative Capacity in Sedentary Adults," *Medicine & Science in Sports & Exercise* 43, no. 10 (2011).

43. David Thivel, et al, "The 24-h Energy Intake of Obese Adolescents is Spontaneously Reduced after Intensive Exercise: A Randomized Controlled Trial in Calorimetric Chambers," *PLoS One* 7, no. 1 (2012): doi:10.1371/journal.pone.0029840.

44. Will Alsop quoted in "Can Architecture Make You Fat?" *The Guardian*, January 2, 2007, http://www.theguardian.com/artanddesign/2007/jan/03/architecture.communities.

45. Phillipe Meyer, Bengt, Kayser, and François Mach, "Stair Use for Cardiovascular Disease Prevention," *European Journal of Cardiovascular Prevention and Rehabilitation* 16, sup. 2 (2009).

46. Sanex Walk for Skin survey reported in "Lazy Brits Spend More than 36 YEARS Sitting On Their Bottoms," *Daily Mail*, April 14, 2008, http://www.dailymail.co.uk/news/article-1015237/Lazy-Brits-spend-36-YEARS-sitting-bottoms.html.

47. Marc T. Hamilton, Deborah G. Hamilton, and Theodore W. Zderic, "Role of Low Energy Expenditure and Sitting in Obesity, Metabolic Syndrome, Type 2 Diabetes, and Cardiovascular Disease," *Diabetes* 56, no. 11 (September 2007).

48. Lawrence D. Frank, Martin A. Andresen, and Thomas L. Schmid, "Obesity Relationships with Community Design, Physical Activity, and Time Spent in Cars," *American Journal of Preventive Medicine* 27, no. 2 (2004).

49. Dena M. Bravata, et al., "Using Pedometers to Increase Physical Activity and Improve Health: A Systematic Review," *Journal of the American Medical Association* 298, no. 19 (November 2007).

50. Alicia J. Crum and Ellen J. Langer, "Mind-Set Matters: exercise and the placebo effect," *Psychological Science* 18, no. 2 (2007).

INDEX

Index

ACKNOWLEDGMENTS

My thanks, as always, go to Dr. Michael Mosley, originator of the 5:2 Diet and a constantly inspiring companion on this remarkable adventure. Thank you, too, to my friends Rebecca Nicolson and Aurea Carpenter, and to the ever-fantastic FastDiet team—Paul Bougourd, Emmie Francis, Klara Zak, Catherine Gibbs, Georgia Vaux, Dr. Sarah Schenker, and Annie Hudson. I'd also like to offer my personal thanks to the many people who have shared their 5:2 stories with us. In the last instance, it is your progress toward health and well-being that underpins all that we do. Closer to home, my family deserves a huge hug for putting up with a mother who is sometimes (but not always) too busy to bake cakes.

Index

Index

Index

the fastbeach diet DAY-BY-DAY PLANNER

YOUR SIX WEEKS STARTS HERE!

Mark out your Fast Days on the chart for the next six weeks—perhaps get yourself a neon highlighter pen to plot the course ahead. Make sure that your diary can accommodate a fast on those days. Clear the decks and make sure you have Fast-friendly food on hand.

Make a note of your starting stats. Measure your start weight—be honest—and your target weight— be realistic. Measure your start BMI and your initial fitness. Tell your family and friends you're doing it. Tell yourself you can do it. Six weeks will disappear in the blink of an eye.

Start weight
....

Target weight
....

Start BMI
....

To measure this, go to thefastdiet.co.uk or download the new Fast Beach Diet app

Strength test: number of push-ups
....

Anybody who finds it hard to do standard push-ups can do modified push-ups, i.e., resting on your elbows rather than on your hands.

Fat %
....

The easiest way to do this is with weighing scales that measure your fat percentage as well as your weight.

Resting heart rate
....

This is to measure your cardio fitness: either use a gadget, or take your pulse for 10 seconds and multiply the result by 6 to get your heart rate per minute.

week 1

> "Take time to deliberate, but when the time for action has arrived, stop thinking and go in."
> *Napoléon Bonaparte*

WHAT TO EXPECT If you've never fasted before, the first Fast Day can be tough. Keep busy. Stay hydrated. Your mission is simple: get through the day, reminding yourself that tomorrow will be easier. Remember, hunger will pass.

Food diary

Date	Fast Day?	Calories eaten	Calories from drinks
1			
2			
3			
4			
5			
6			
7			

Weigh-in after Fast Day 1 _____   Waist measurement day 7 _____   Fat % day 7

Weigh-in after Fast Day 2 _____   BMI day 7 _____   _____

Exercise diary

Date	Cardio completed	Strength training
1		
2		
3		
4		
5		
6		
7		

Strength test day 7 _____   How are you feeling? _____

Resting heart rate day 7 _____

week 2

WHAT TO EXPECT You've knocked off two full-on Fast Days and know the ropes now. Stay focused. Your Fast Days should start getting easier from now on.

Food diary

Date	Fast Day?	Calories eaten	Calories from drinks
1			
2			
3			
4			
5			
6			
7			

Weigh-in after Fast Day 1 _____

Weigh-in after Fast Day 2 _____

Waist measurement day 7 _____

BMI day 7 _____

Fat % day 7 _____

Exercise diary

Date	Cardio completed	Strength training
1		
2		
3		
4		
5		
6		
7		

Strength test day 7 _____

Resting heart rate day 7 _____

How are you feeling? _____

week 3

"If we are facing in the right direction, all we have to do is keep on walking."
Buddhist saying

WHAT TO EXPECT By the end of this week, you'll be halfway through, so take heart. If you're seeing movement on the scales, use that to bounce you through these middle weeks. As your fitness increases, step up your HIT by increasing resistance or reps.

Food diary

Date	Fast Day?	Calories eaten	Calories from drinks
1			
2			
3			
4			
5			
6			
7			

Weigh-in after Fast Day 1

Weigh-in after Fast Day 2

Waist measurement day 7

BMI day 7

Fat % day 7

Exercise diary

Date	Cardio completed	Strength training
1		
2		
3		
4		
5		
6		
7		

Strength test day 7

Resting heart rate day 7

How are you feeling?

week 4

WHAT TO EXPECT New habits are beginning to form. Congratulate yourself, reward yourself and tell people about your achievements. If you're feeling a bit lost, go on the forums (ours is at www.thefastdiet.co.uk) for support, advice, and a group hug.

Food diary

Date	Fast Day?	Calories eaten	Calories from drinks
1			
2			
3			
4			
5			
6			
7			

Weigh-in after Fast Day 1

Weigh-in after Fast Day 2

Waist measurement day 7

BMI day 7

Fat % day 7

Exercise diary

Date	Cardio completed	Strength training
1		
2		
3		
4		
5		
6		
7		

Strength test day 7

Resting heart rate day 7

How are you feeling?

week 5

"Success is a staircase, not a doorway."
Dottie Walters

WHAT TO EXPECT You've been doing the FastBeach Diet for over a month now, and you may find that your appetite and taste for food has started to change. Check your portion sizes: Have they gotten smaller? If you've managed without alcohol, your body will have started to gain measurable benefit. Not long now till you can celebrate . . .

Food diary

Date	Fast Day?	Calories eaten	Calories from drinks
1			
2			
3			
4			
5			
6			
7			

Weigh-in after Fast Day 1 _____ Waist measurement day 7 _____ Fat % day 7

Weigh-in after Fast Day 2 _____ BMI day 7 _____

Exercise diary

Date	Cardio completed	Strength training
1		
2		
3		
4		
5		
6		
7		

Strength test day 7 _____ How are you feeling? _____

Resting heart rate day 7 _____

week 6

"When you reach the end of your rope, tie a knot in it and hang on."
Thomas Jefferson

WHAT TO EXPECT The final week of the FastBeach Diet: The habits and techniques you're instilling now will help you in the days ahead as you resume your 5:2. Occasional treats will be back on the menu. Just one more week of tough love and you're done.

Food diary

Date	Fast Day?	Calories eaten	Calories from drinks
1			
2			
3			
4			
5			
6			
7			

Weigh-in after Fast Day 1 _____

Weigh-in after Fast Day 2 _____

Waist measurement day 7 _____

BMI day 7 _____

Fat % day 7 _____

Exercise diary

Date	Cardio completed	Strength training
1		
2		
3		
4		
5		
6		
7		

Strength test day 7 _____

Resting heart rate day 7 _____

Congratulations! You should be feeling great...

The FastBeach Diet Checklist

Tighten up on Fast Days

Go to 4:3

Try 2-to-2

Extend your Fasting Window

Be fast-idious about your Fast Day calorie quota

Toughen up on non-Fast Days

Cut out alcohol
Or reduce alcohol intake

Shift your eating habits
Avoid refined carbs
Cook at home when you can
Cut back on treats
Choose unpackaged food
Cut the 50/50s
Move towards a Mediterranean diet
Cook to suit the summertime:
    Grill and barbecue
    Choose raw foods
    Embrace Japanese food
    Eat more fish
    Choose soup
    Implement the Rule of Three-
    Quarters
    Have a Meatless Monday
    Go part-veggie and make meat a
    once-a-week treat

Watch what you drink
Junk the juice
Drop the soda
Choose the right coffee

Sleep well
Get a good eight hours in

Tune in on any day

Cultivate mindfulness around food
Don't eat on autopilot
Stop when you're satisfied, not when
you're full

Give yourself visual clues
Smaller plates, smaller glasses, smaller
portions
Wait before you eat and go slow
Keep a food diary

Tackle temptation
Use the Proximity Principle
Make healthy foods available
Don't eat from the box
Don't get distracted
Use site-specific aversion therapy

Get a handle on habit
Undermine the status quo with
deliberate practice
Make specific commitments, not
vague ones
Give yourself positive feedback
Keep the commitment small
Know your triggers
Work on your willpower
    Don't feel bad, feel good
    Say "I will," not "I won't"
    Reframe the motivator
    Find a goal role model

Add exercise

Introduce HIT three days a week

**Introduce strength training two days
a week**

Make it happen
Put on your workout clothes in the
morning
Keep your workout shoes by the door
Write a pledge, be specific
Make a list of excuses; make a list of
solutions
Monitor your progress
Use your environment

Get up, get out, get going
Stand up and walk around at least once
every hour
Have a car-free week
Tell people
Find a friend to exercise with
Get a gadget—
    use the FastBeach Diet app

If you would prefer to print a larger format version of this planner in A4, or if you would like to give one to a friend, please go to: http://thefastdiet.co.uk/wp-content/uploads/2014/04/FB-PLANNER.pdf